Pulmonary Pathophysiology
—*the essentials*
3rd edition

Pulmonary
Pathophysiology
—*the essentials*
3rd edition

John B. West, M.D., Ph.D.

Professor of Medicine and Physiology
University of California, San Diego
School of Medicine
La Jolla, California

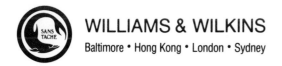

WILLIAMS & WILKINS
Baltimore • Hong Kong • London • Sydney

Editor: John N. Gardner
Associate Editor: Linda Napora
Copy Editor: Barbara Farabaugh
Design: JoAnne Janowiak
Illustration Planning: Wayne Hubbel
Production: Raymond E. Reter

Printed in the United States of America

First edition, 1977
Second edition, 1982
Portuguese translation, 1978
Spanish translation, 1979
Italian translation, 1981
Japanese translation, 1981 and 1983
Dutch translation, 1981

Library of Congress Cataloging-in-Publication Data

West, John B. (John Burnard)
  Pulmonary pathophysiology.

  Bibliography: p.
  Includes index.
1 1. Lungs—Diseases. 2. Pulmonary function tests. 3. Physiology, Pathological. I. Title. [DNLM: 1. Lung—physiopathology. WF 600 W514p]
RC732.W47 1987   616.2'407   86–19111
ISBN 0-683-08941-2

90 91
10 9 8 7 6 5

To R.B.W.

Preface to the 3rd Edition

This text has been completely revised and brought up to date in a number of areas including the pathophysiology of asthma, pulmonary edema and pulmonary embolism, positive end-expiratory pressure, respiratory muscle fatigue, and acute respiratory failure. However, the length of the book has been kept nearly the same by careful pruning of other areas. A number of readers have written about various points in the book; these comments are much appreciated. A set of audio tapes and slides to supplement the material in the book is available from Audio Visual Medical Marketing, Inc., 235 Park Avenue South, New York, NY 10003.

Preface to the 1st Edition

This book is written as a companion to *Respiratory Physiology— The Essentials* and is about the function of the diseased as opposed to the normal lung. It is primarily intended for medical students in their second and subsequent years. However, a concise, amply illustrated account of respiratory function in disease may prove useful to the increasingly large number of physicians and paramedical personnel who come into contact with respiratory patients. These include anesthesiologists, cardiologists, intensive care personnel, and respiratory therapists.

Many medical schools are constantly trying to emphasize the relevance of the basic science of the first two years to the practice of medicine. Respiratory function can be a model for this. A discussion of a patient with asthma, for example, can cover the basic physiology of the airways, blood gases and lung volumes quickly and painlessly. It is hoped that this little book will be helpful in such a course.

This book emphasizes the relations between structure and function in the diseased lung. Indeed the reader will find more anatomic pathology than he might expect in a book about pathophysiology. But

Editor's note: The illustrations credited on page x have been renumbered in this 3rd edition. The current designations of the figures are as follows: Academic Press, Figure 4.5*B*; *American Journal of Medicine*, Figure 7.4; American Lung Association, Figure 8.2; American Physiological Society, Figures 3.2, 4.9, 5.1, and 10.6; Blackwell Scientific, Figures 2.1 and 10.6; British Medical Association, Figure 3.3; Churchill-Livingstone, Figures 4.2, 4.3, and 4.5*A*, Marcel Dekker, Figure 9.3; McGraw Hill, Figure 4.4; *New England Journal of Medicine*, Figure 3.4; New York Academy of Sciences, Figure 7.7; Rockefeller University Press, Figure 2.10; W. B. Saunders Co., Figures 2.7, 3.1, 4.6, 4.7, 4.12, 4.16, and 6.3; and Williams & Wilkins, Figures 5.3 and 9.5.

Information concerning audio tapes is now available from Audio Visual Medical Marketing, Inc., 235 Park Avenue South, New York, NY 10003.

function cannot be properly understood without a knowledge of structure. It is assumed that students who read this book are also exposed to teaching in pathology.

Naturally such a concise book covering such a wide area must be dogmatic. However, the reader will find a full discussion of disputed issues in the references and reading list at the end of the book. I would be grateful for any comments on the selection of material and factual errors. A set of audiotapes with slides is available to supplement this book.*

Several colleagues have read parts of the manuscript and have suggested improvements. They include: Drs. Arend Bouhuys, Benjamin Burrows, David H. Dail, Ronald Dueck, James C. Hogg, Norman Jones, D. F. C. Muir, John F. Murray, Norman C. Staub, and Peter D. Wagner, Drs. Paul J. Friedman and Michael P. Hlastala helped with the selection of radiographs and Dr. Peter D. Wagner assisted with the diagrams. I am indebted to all of them. I would also like to acknowledge the secretarial assistance of Mrs. Elizabeth Silva and the friendly help of Mr. James Gallagher and others on the staff of The Williams & Wilkins Co.

The publishers of the following journals and books kindly gave permission for the use of material. The sources are cited in the figure captions: Academic Press Inc., New York, Figure 34B; *American Journal of Medicine*, Figure 68; American Lung Association, Figure 73; American Physiological Society, Figures 26, 39, 49, and 87; Blackwell Scientific Publications, Oxford, Figures 12 and 88; British Medical Association, London, Figure 27; Churchill-Livingstone Publishers, London, Figures 31, 32, and 34A, Marcel Dekker Inc., New York, Figure 77; McGraw Hill, New York, Figure 33; *New England Journal of Medicine*, Boston, Figure 28; New York Academy of Sciences, New York, Figure 71; Rockefeller University Press, New York, Figure 21; W. B. Saunders Co., Philadelphia, Figures 18, 25, 35, 36, 42, 45, and 59; and The Williams & Wilkins Co, Baltimore, Figures 51 and 79.

---

* Information from John B. West, M.D., Ph.D., Department of Medicine, University of California, San Diego, La Jolla, California 92093.

Contents

CONTENTS

SECTION ONE

LUNG FUNCTION TESTS AND WHAT THEY MEAN

1. Ventilation
2. Gas exchange
3. Other tests

We learn how diseased lungs work by doing pulmonary function tests. Accordingly, this section is devoted to a description of the most important tests and their interpretation. It is assumed that the reader is familiar with the basic physiology of the lung as contained in the companion volume, J. B. West: *Respiratory Physiology—The Essentials*, ed. 3. Baltimore, Williams & Wilkins, 1985.

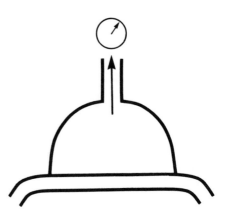

chapter 1

Ventilation

The simplest test of lung function is a forced expiration. It is also one of the most informative tests and it requires a minimum of equipment and trivial calculations. The majority of patients with lung disease have an abnormal forced expiration and very often the information obtained from this test is useful in their management. In spite of this, the test is not used as often as it should be. For example, it can be valuable in detecting early airway disease, an extremely common and important condition.

TESTS OF VENTILATORY CAPACITY

Forced Expiratory Volume

The *forced expiratory volume* (FEV) is the volume of gas exhaled in *one second* by a forced expiration from full inspiration. The *vital capacity* is the *total* volume of gas that can be exhaled after a full inspiration.

A simple way of making these measurements is shown in Figure 1.1. The patient is comfortably seated in front of a spirometer having a low resistence. He breathes in maximally and then exhales as hard

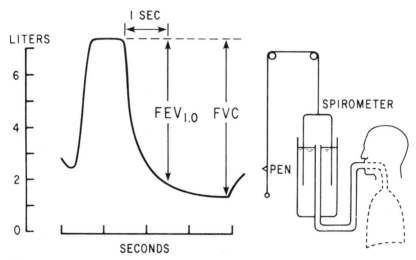

Figure 1.1. Measurement of forced expiratory volume ($FEV_{1.0}$) and vital capacity (FVC).

and as far as he can. As the spirometer bell moves up, the kymograph pen moves down, thus indicating the expired volume against time.

Figure 1.2A shows a normal tracing. It can be seen that the volume exhaled in 1 sec was 4.0 liters and the total volume exhaled was 5.0 liters. These two volumes are therefore the forced expiratory volume in 1 sec ($FEV_{1.0}$) and the vital capacity. The vital capacity measured with a forced expiration may be less than that measured with a slower exhalation, so that the term forced vital capacity (FVC) is generally used. Note that the normal ratio of $FEV_{1.0}$ to FVC is about 80%. (See Appendix for normal values.)

Figure 1.2B shows the type of tracing obtained from a patient with chronic obstructive lung disease. Note that the rate at which the air was exhaled was much slower, so that only 1.3 liters were blown out in the first second. In addition, the total volume exhaled was only 3.1 liters. $FEV_{1.0}$/FVC was reduced to 42%. These figures are typical of an *obstructive* pattern.

Contrast this pattern with that of Figure 1.2C, which shows the type of tracing obtained from a patient with pulmonary fibrosis. Here the vital capacity was reduced to 3.1 liters, but a large percentage (90%) was exhaled in the first second. These figures mean *restrictive* disease.

If the equipment shown in Figure 1.1 is used, the spirometer should

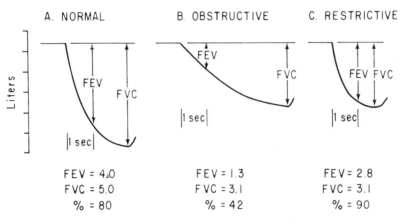

Figure 1.2. Normal, obstructive, and restrictive patterns of a forced expiration.

be light with a wide diameter, and the tubing should have a low resistance so that the spirometer can respond rapidly. Dry spirometers using the bellows principle are also available and are convenient for measurements at the bedside. Sometimes they provide a graph which can be filed with the patient's chart. Various electronic spirometers are also on the market, but these should be carefully calibrated.

The patient should loosen any tight clothing and the mouthpiece should be at a convenient height. One accepted procedure is to allow two practice blows and then record three good test breaths. The highest $FEV_{1.0}$ and FVC from these three breaths are then used. The volumes should be converted to body temperature and pressure (see Appendix). Further practical details can be found elsewhere (1).

The test is often of value in assessing the efficacy of bronchodilator drugs. If reversible airway obstruction is suspected, the test should be carried out before and after administering the drug (for example, 1% isoproterenol by nebulizer for 3 min). Both the $FEV_{1.0}$ and FVC usually increase in a patient with bronchospasm.

Forced Expiratory Flow ($FEF_{25-75\%}$)

This index is calculated from the tracing in Figure 1.3. The middle half (by volume) of the total expiration is marked and its duration is measured. The $FEF_{25-75\%}$ is the volume in liters divided by the time in seconds (2).

The correlation between $FEF_{25-75\%}$ and FEV is generally close in

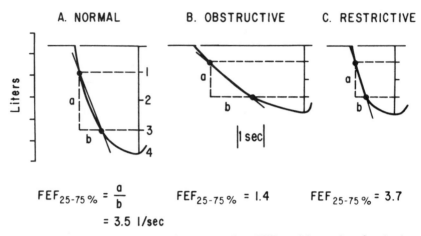

Figure 1.3.   Calculation of forced expiratory flow ($FEF_{25-75\%}$) from a forced expiration.

patients with obstructive lung disease. The changes in $FEF_{25-75\%}$ are often more striking, but the range of normal values is greater.

Interpretation of Tests of Forced Expiration

In some respects, the lungs and thorax can be regarded as a simple air pump (Figure 1.4). The output of such a pump depends on the stroke volume, the resistance of the airways, and the forced applied to the piston. The last factor is relatively unimportant in a forced expiration, as we shall presently see.

The *vital capacity* (or forced vital capacity) is a measure of the stroke volume, and any reduction in it will affect the ventilatory capacity. Causes of stroke volume reduction include diseases of the thoracic cage, such as kyphoscoliosis, ankylosing spondylitis, and acute injuries; diseases affecting the nerve supply to the respiratory muscles or the muscles themselves, such as poliomyelitis or muscular dystrophy; abnormalities of the pleural cavity, such as pneumothorax or pleural thickening; pathology in the lung itself, such as fibrosis, which reduces its distensibility, space-occupying lesions such as cysts, or an increased pulmonary blood volume, as in left heart failure. In addition, there are diseases of the airways which cause them to close prematurely during expiration, thus limiting the volume which can be exhaled. This occurs in asthma and bronchitis.

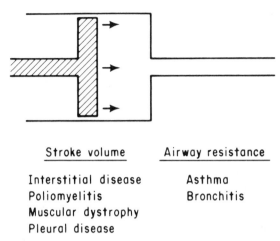

Stroke volume	Airway resistance
Interstitial disease	Asthma
Poliomyelitis	Bronchitis
Muscular dystrophy	
Pleural disease	

Figure 1.4. Simple model of factors which may reduce the ventilatory capacity. The stroke volume may be reduced by diseases of the lung parenchyma, pleura, or respiratory muscle. Airway resistance is increased in asthma and bronchitis.

The *forced expiratory volume* (and related indices such as the $FEF_{25-75\%}$) is affected by the airway resistance during forced expiration. Any increase in resistance will reduce the ventilatory capacity. Causes include bronchoconstriction as in asthma or following the inhalation of irritants such as cigarette smoke, structural changes in the airways as in chronic bronchitis, obstructions within the airways such as an inhaled foreign body or excess bronchial secretions, and destructive processes in the lung parenchyma which interfere with the radial traction that normally supports the airways.

While the simple model of Figure 1.4 serves as an introduction to the factors limiting the ventilatory capacity of the diseased lung, we need to refine the model to obtain a better understanding. For example, the airways are actually *inside* the pump, not *outside*, as shown in Figure 1.4. Useful additional information comes from the flow-volume curve.

Flow-Volume Curve

If we record flow rate and volume during a maximal forced expiration, we obtain a pattern like that shown in Figure 1.5A. A curious feature of the flow-volume curve is that it is virtually impossible to get outside it. For example, if we begin by exhaling slowly and then exert maxi-

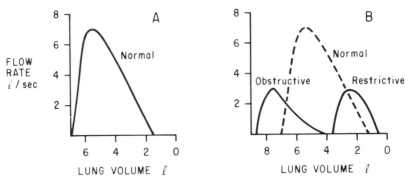

Figure 1.5.   Flow-volume curves. (*A*) Normal. (*B*) Obstructive and restrictive patterns.

mum effort, the flow rate will increase to the envelope but not beyond. Clearly, something very powerful is limiting the maximum flow rate at a given volume. This factor is dynamic compression of the airways.

Figure 1.5*B* shows typical patterns found in obstructive and restrictive lung disease. In obstructive diseases such as chronic bronchitis and emphysema, the maximal expiration typically begins and ends at abnormally high lung volumes and the flow rates are much lower than normal. In addition, the curve may have a scooped out appearance. By contrast, patients with restrictive disease such as interstitial fibrosis operate at low lung volumes. Their flow envelope is flattened compared with normal, but if flow rate is related to lung volume, the flow is seen to be higher than normal (Fig. 1.5*B*). Note that the figure shows absolute lung volumes, though these cannot be obtained from a forced expiration. They require an additional measurement of residual volume.

To understand these patterns, consider the pressures inside and outside the airways* (Figure 1.6). Before inspiration (*A*), the pressures in the mouth, airways and alveoli are all atmospheric because there is no flow. Intrapleural pressure is, say, 5 cm water below atmospheric pressure, and we assume that the same pressure exists outside the airways (though this is an oversimplification). Thus, the pressure difference expanding the airways is 5 cm water. At the beginning of inspiration (*B*), all pressures fall and the pressure difference holding

---

* See J. B. West: *Respiratory Physiology—The Essentials*, ed. 3, p. 106. Baltimore, Williams & Wilkins, 1985.

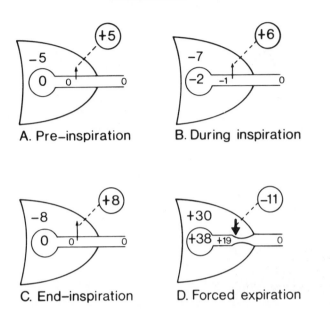

Figure 1.6. Diagram explaining dynamic compression of the airways during a forced expiration. (See text for details.)

the airways open increases to 6 cm water. At the end of inspiration (*C*), this pressure is 8 cm water.

Early in a forced expiration (*D*), both intrapleural and alveolar pressures rise greatly. The pressure at some point in the airways increases, but not as much as alveolar pressure because of the pressure drop caused by flow. Under these circumstances we have a pressure difference of 11 cm water tending to *close* the airways. Airway compression occurs, and now flow is determined by the difference between alveolar pressure and the pressure outside the airways at the collapse point (Starling resistor effect). Note that this pressure difference (8 cm water in *D*) is the static recoil pressure of the lung and is dependent only on lung volume and compliance. It is *independent* of expiratory effort.

How then can we explain the abnormal patterns in Figure 1.5*B*? In the patient with chronic bronchitis and emphysema, the low flow rate in relation to lung volume is caused by several factors. There may be thickening of the walls of the airways and excessive secretions in the lumen because of bronchitis; both increase the flow resistance. The number of small airways may be reduced because of destruction of lung tissue. Also, the patient may have a reduced static recoil pressure (even though lung volume is greatly increased) because of breakdown of elastic alveolar walls. Finally, the normal support offered to the airways by the traction of the surrounding parenchyma is probably impaired because of loss of alveolar walls, and the airways therefore collapse more easily than they should. These factors are considered in more detail in Chapter 4.

The patient with interstitial fibrosis has normal (or high) flow rates in relation to lung volume because his lung static recoil pressures are high and the caliber of his airways may be normal (or even increased) at a given lung volume. However, because of the greatly reduced compliance of the lung, the lung volumes are very small and absolute flow rates are therefore reduced.

This analysis shows that Figure 1.4 is a considerable oversimplification and that the forced expiratory volume which seems so straightforward at first sight is affected by both the airways and the lung parenchyma. Thus, the terms "obstructive" and "restrictive" conceal a good deal of pathophysiology.

Partitioning of Flow Resistance from the Flow-Volume Curve

When the airways collapse during a forced expiration, the flow rate is determined by the resistance of the airways up to the point of collapse (Figure 1.7). Beyond this point, the resistance of the airways is immaterial. Collapse occurs at (or near) the point where the pressure inside the airways is equal to the intrapleural pressure (sometimes called the *equal pressure point*). This is believed to be in the vicinity of the lobar bronchi early in a forced expiration. However, as lung volume reduces and the airways narrow, their resistance increases. As a result pressure is lost more rapidly and the collapse point moves into more distal airways. Thus, late in forced expiration, flow is increasingly determined by the properties of the small peripheral airways.

These peripheral airways (say less than 2 mm diameter) normally contribute less than 20% of the total airway resistance. Therefore, changes in them are difficult to detect and they constitute a "silent zone." However, it is likely that some of the earliest changes in chronic obstructive lung disease occur in these small airways, and therefore

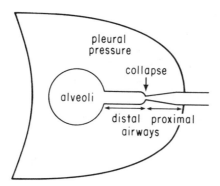

Figure 1.7. When dynamic compression of the airways occurs during a forced expiration, only the resistance of the airways distal to the point of collapse (upstream segment) determines the flow rate. In the last stages of a forced vital capacity, only the peripheral small airways are distal to the collapsed point and therefore determine the flow.

the maximum flow rate late in a forced expiration is often taken to reflect peripheral airway resistance.

Maximum Flows from the Flow-Volume Curve

Maximum flow ($\dot{V}_{max}$) is frequently measured after 50% ($\dot{V}_{max_{50\%}}$) or 75% ($\dot{V}_{max_{75\%}}$) of the vital capacity has been exhaled. Figure 1.8 shows an example of the abnormal pattern typically seen in chronic obstructive lung disease. The later in expiration that the flow is measured, the more the measurement reflects the resistance of the very small airways. Some studies have shown abnormalities in the $\dot{V}_{max_{75\%}}$ when other indices of a forced expiration such as the FEV or $FEF_{25-75\%}$ were normal.

Inspiratory Flow-Volume Curve

The flow-volume curve is also often measured during inspiration. This curve is not affected by dynamic compression of the airways because the pressures during inspiration always expand the bronchi (Figure 1.6). However, the curve is sometimes useful in detecting upper airway obstruction, which flattens the curve because maximum flow is limited. Causes include glottic or tracheal stenosis and tracheal narrowing as a result of a compressing neoplasm. The expiratory flow-volume curve is also flattened by upper airway obstruction.

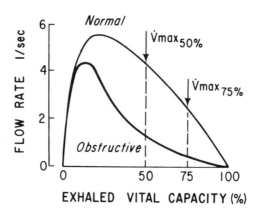

Figure 1.8.   Example of a flow-volume curve in chronic obstructive lung disease. Note the scooped-out appearance. The *arrows* show the maximum expiratory flow after 50% and 75% of the vital capacity have been exhaled.

Flow-Volume Curve during Helium Breathing

Another technique for determining the resistance of small airways from the flow-volume curve is to use a gas of low density. If a mixture of 80% helium and 20% oxygen is breathed, the pressure drop in the large airways is considerably reduced. This is because the flow there is turbulent and the pressure drop is therefore determined in part by the density of the gas. By contrast, the pressure drop in the small airways where flow is chiefly laminar is little affected. Therefore, in a patient whose peripheral airways are partially obstructed, the change in the flow-volume curve when helium-oxygen is breathed is less than in normal subjects. Various indices for assessing the response of the curve have been described (3). These include the flow rate at 50% of the vital capacity, and the lung volume at which the air and helium-oxygen curves become superimposed.

Airway and Parenchymal Components of the Flow-Volume Curve

We have seen that the forced expiratory volume may be reduced by an increase in airway resistance or a reduced elastic recoil pressure because of parenchymal disease. Is there any way to distinguish between these two factors? One way is to plot the maximum flow rate against the elastic recoil pressure as shown in Figure 1.9. This cannot

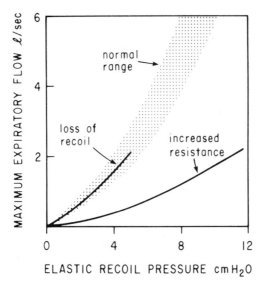

Figure 1.9. Interpretation of a reduced maximum expiratory flow rate. If this is caused solely by parenchymal disease, the normal relationship between maximum flow and recoil pressure is retained. However, increased airway resistance disturbs the relationship.

be done from a forced expiration alone because we also need to record esophageal pressure (as a measure of intrapleural pressure) under static conditions at the various lung volumes of the vital capacity. But the method is described here because it throws light on the interpretation of the flow-volume curve.

If the airways are normal and the reduced flow rate is caused solely by parenchymal disease, the relationship between flow and elastic recoil pressure is unchanged. This pattern is seen (very nearly) in patients thought to have emphysema without bronchitis. On the other hand, if the airways are diseased but the parenchyma is normal, the curve departs from the normal range. This pattern is seen in patients with bronchial asthma (Figure 4.9).

Transit Time Analysis

Another way of analyzing a forced expiration is to compute the average time required for a gas particle to leave the lung (transit time). Additional indices such as the standard deviation and skewness of the transit times can also be derived. An advantage of these measurements is that they are independent of lung size, and some data suggest that the procedures give a sensitive indicator of airway disease.

Perspective on the Measurement of Flow-Volume Curves

The physiological basis of flow-volume curves has been described in some detail because this information is required for a clear understanding of the simple tests of forced expiratory volume and maximum midexpiratory flow. This does not mean that flow-volume curves need be measured routinely; this is especially true of the variants such as the flow-volume curve during helium-oxygen breathing. In many instances the simple forced expiration test is sufficient, and indeed it should be exploited more than it is.

TESTS OF UNEVEN VENTILATION

Single Breath Nitrogen Test

The tests described so far measure ventilatory capacity. The single breath nitrogen test measures inequality of ventilation. This is a somewhat different topic but it is conveniently described here.

Suppose a patient takes a single vital capacity inspiration of oxygen and then exhales slowly to residual volume. If we measure the nitrogen concentration at the mouthpiece with a rapid nitrogen analyzer, we record a pattern as shown in Figure 1.10. Four phases can be recognized. In the first, which is very short, pure oxygen is exhaled from the upper airways and the nitrogen concentration is zero. In the second phase there is a rapid rise in nitrogen concentration as the anatomic dead space is washed out by alveolar gas. This phase is also short.

The third phase consists of alveolar gas, and the tracing is almost flat in normal subjects. This portion is often known as the alveolar plateau. In patients with uneven ventilation the third phase steadily rises and the slope is a measure of the inequality of ventilation. It is expressed as the percentage increase in nitrogen concentration per liter of expired volume; the range of normal values is given in the Appendix. In carrying out this test, care should be taken to keep the expiratory flow rate less than 0.5 liters/sec in order to reduce the variability of the results.

The reasons for the rise in nitrogen concentration in phase 3 are not fully understood. Apparently there are some regions of lung which

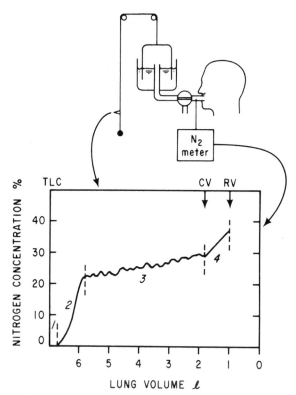

Figure 1.10.   Single breath nitrogen test of uneven ventilation. Note the four phases of the expired tracing. *CV*, closing volume. (See text for details.)

are poorly ventilated and therefore receive relatively little of the breath of oxygen. These areas will therefore have a relatively high concentration of nitrogen because there is less oxygen to dilute this gas. Also these poorly ventilated regions tend to empty last.

Three possible mechanisms are shown in Figure 1.11. In *A*, the region is poorly ventilated because of partial obstruction of its airway, and because of this high resistance the region empties late. In fact, the rate of emptying of such a region is determined by its time constant, which is given by the product of its airway resistance (R) and compliance (C). The larger the time constant (RC), the longer it will take to empty. This mechanism is known as *parallel* inequality of ventilation.

Figure 1.11*B* shows a different mechanism known as *series* inequality. Here there is a dilation of peripheral airspaces causing differences

Inequality of Ventilation

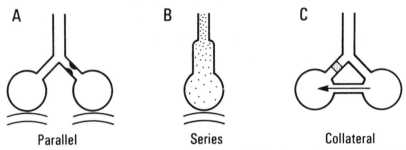

A   B   C

Parallel   Series   Collateral

Figure 1.11. Three mechanisms of uneven ventilation. In parallel inequality (A), flow to regions with long time constants is reduced. In series inequality (B), dilatation of a small airway may result in impaired diffusion along a terminal lung unit. Collateral ventilation (C) may also cause series inequality.

of ventilation *along* the air passages of a lung unit. In this context we should recall that inspired gas reaches the terminal bronchioles by convective flow, that is, like water running through a hose, but its subsequent movement to the alveoli is chiefly accomplished by diffusion within the airways. Normally the distances are so short that nearly complete equilibration of gas concentrations is quickly established. However, if there is enlargement of the small airways, as occurs for example, in centrilobular emphysema (Figure 4.4), the concentration of inspired gas in the most distal airways remains low. Again these poorly ventilated regions will empty last.

Figure 1.11C shows another form of series inequality which occurs when some lung units receive their inspired gas from neighboring units rather than the large airways. This is known as collateral ventilation and appears to be an important process in obstructive lung diseases.

There is still uncertainty about the relative importance of parallel and series inequality, but it is likely that both operate to some extent in normal subjects and in a much exaggerated form in patients with obstructive lung disease. Whatever the mechanism, the single breath nitrogen test is a simple, rapid, and reliable way of measuring the degree of uneven ventilation in the lung. This is increased in most obstructive and many restrictive types of lung disease (see Chapters 4 and 5).

Closing Volume

Toward the end of the vital capacity expiration shown in Figure 1.10 there is an abrupt rise in nitrogen concentration, which signals the onset of airway closure or phase 4. The volume of phase 4 is called the *closing volume*, and the closing volume plus the residual volume is known as the *closing capacity*. In practice the onset of phase 4 is obtained by drawing a straight line through the alveolar plateau (phase 3) and noting the last point of departure of the nitrogen tracing from this line.

Unfortunately it is seldom that the junction between phases 3 and 4 is as clear-cut as in Figure 1.10, and there is considerable variation of this volume when repeated measurements are made on the same patient. The test is most useful in the presence of small amounts of disease, because severe disease distorts the tracing so much that the closing volume cannot be identified.

The mechanism of the onset of phase 4 is still disputed, but much evidence suggests that it is caused by closure of small airways in the lowest part of the lung. At residual volume just before the single breath of oxygen, the nitrogen concentration is virtually uniform throughout the lung, but the basal alveoli are much smaller than the apical alveoli because of distortion of the lung by its weight. Indeed the lowest portions are compressed so much that the small airways in the region of the respiratory bronchioles are closed. However, at the end of a vital capacity inspiration, all the alveoli are approximately the same size. Thus, the nitrogen at the base is diluted much more than that of the apex by the breath of oxygen.

During the subsequent expiration, the upper and lower zones empty together and the expired nitrogen concentration is nearly constant (Figure 1.10). But as soon as dependent airways begin to close, the higher nitrogen concentration in the upper zones preferentially affects the expired concentration, causing an abrupt rise. Moreover, as airway closure proceeds up the lung, the expired nitrogen progressively increases.

The volume at which airways close is very age-dependent, being as low as 10% of the vital capacity in young normal subjects but increasing to 40%, that is, approximately the FRC, at about the age of 65 years. There is some evidence that the test is sensitive to small amounts of disease. For example, apparently healthy cigarette smokers sometimes have increased closing volumes when their ventilatory capacity is normal.

Other Tests of Uneven Ventilation

Uneven ventilation can also be measured by a multibreath nitrogen washout during oxygen breathing. Topographical inequality of ventilation can be determined using radioactive xenon. The present chapter is confined to single breath tests; these other measurements are taken up in Chapter 3.

Tests of Early Airway Disease

There has been great interest in the possible use of some of the tests described in this chapter to identify patients with early airway disease. The reason for this is that once a patient develops the full picture of chronic obstructive lung disease, the results of treatment are generally disappointing. The hope is that by identifying disease at an early stage, its progression can be slowed, for example, by the patient stopping cigarette smoking.

Among the tests that have been examined in this context are the FEV, $FEF_{25-75\%}$, $\dot{V}_{max_{50\%}}$, and $\dot{V}_{max_{75\%}}$, the flow-volume curve during helium breathing, and the closing volume. Assessment of these tests is difficult because it depends on prospective studies and large control groups. Although work continues, it is clear that the original test of FEV remains one of the most reliable and valuable tests. While more sophisticated tests should clearly be investigated, measuring the FEV and FVC remains mandatory.

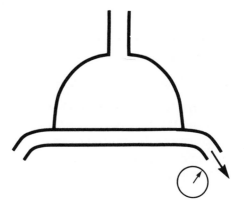

chapter 2

Gas Exchange

Chapter 1 dealt with the simplest test of lung function: the forced expiration. In addition we looked briefly at other single breath tests of uneven ventilation. In this chapter we turn to the most important measurement in the management of respiratory failure: arterial blood gases. Another test of gas exchange, the diffusing capacity, is also discussed.

BLOOD GASES

Arterial P_{O_2}

Measurement

It is often essential to know the partial pressure of oxygen in the arterial blood of acutely ill patients. With modern blood gas electrodes, the measurement of arterial P_{O_2} is relatively simple, and the test should be available in all hospitals where patients with respiratory failure are managed.

Arterial blood is usually taken by puncture of a brachial, radial, or femoral artery. A single sample is often withdrawn; alternatively a

19

small catheter can be left in the artery and samples taken as required. The dead space of the syringe should be filled with dilute heparin, and ideally the blood should be analyzed within a few minutes. If this is not possible, the syringe should be placed in a beaker of ice to slow down the metabolism of the blood.

Arterial P_{O_2} is measured with a polarographic oxygen electrode (Figure 2.1). The principle is that if a small voltage (0.6 volt) is applied to a platinum electrode immersed in a buffer solution, the current which flows is proportional to the P_{O_2}. In practice the buffer is separated from the blood by a semipermeable membrane through which oxygen diffuses. Oxygen is consumed by the electrode; consequently, the measured P_{O_2} falls with time. The fall is fastest when the P_{O_2} is high. The electrode is calibrated with gas or with a solution of known P_{O_2} (4).

Normal Values

The normal value for arterial P_{O_2} in young adults averages about 95 mm Hg, with a range of about 85–100. The normal value falls steadily with age, and the average is about 85 mm Hg at age 60 years (see

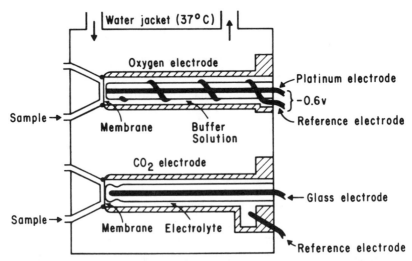

Figure 2.1. Oxygen and carbon dioxide electrodes. In both instances the blood sample is separated from the electrode by a semipermeable membrane. The electrodes are connected to an amplifier which reads P_{O_2} and P_{CO_2} directly. (Modified from J. E. Cotes: *Lung Function*, ed. 4. Oxford, Blackwell, 1979 (4).)

Appendix). The cause of the fall in P_{O_2} is probably increasing ventilation-perfusion inequality (see below).

Whenever we read a report of an arterial P_{O_2} we should have the oxygen dissociation curve at the back of our minds. Figure 2.2 reminds us of two anchor points on the normal curve—arterial blood (P_{O_2} 100, O_2 saturation 97%) and mixed venous blood (P_{O_2} 40, O_2 saturation 75%). Also, we should recall that above 60 mm Hg the curve is fairly flat and cyanosis is probably undetectable. The curve is shifted to the right by an increase in temperature and P_{CO_2} and a fall in pH (these all occur in exercising muscle where enhanced unloading of O_2 is advantageous). The curve is also shifted to the right by an increase in 2,3-diphosphoglycerate (DPG) inside the red cells, which occurs as a result of prolonged hypoxia, for example, in chronic lung disease or cyanotic heart disease. An increased concentration may also occur in anemia.

Causes of Hypoxemia

There are four primary causes of a reduced P_{O_2} in arterial blood:

1. Hypoventilation

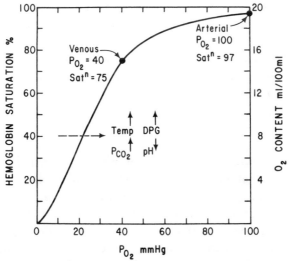

Figure 2.2. Anchor points of the oxygen dissociation curve. The curve is shifted to the right by an increase in temperature, P_{CO_2} and 2,3-DPG and a fall in pH. The oxygen content scale is based on a hemoglobin concentration of 14.5 g/100 ml.

2. Diffusion impairment
3. Shunt
4. Ventilation-perfusion inequality

A fifth cause, reduction of inspired P_{O_2}, such as during residence at high altitude or breathing a mixture of low oxygen concentration, is only seen in special circumstances.

Hypoventilation. This means that the volume of fresh gas going to the alveoli per unit time (alveolar ventilation) is reduced. If the resting oxygen consumption is not correspondingly reduced, this inevitably results in hypoxemia. Hypoventilation is commonly caused by diseases outside the lungs; indeed, very often the lungs are normal.

Two cardinal physiological features of hypoventilation should be emphasized. First, it *always* causes an increased arterial P_{CO_2}, and this is a valuable diagnostic feature. Indeed the relationship between the arterial P_{CO_2} and the level of alveolar ventilation in the normal lung is a very simple one:

$$P_{CO_2} = \frac{\dot{V}_{CO_2}}{\dot{V}_A} \cdot K \qquad [1]$$

where $\dot{V}_{CO_2}$ is the CO_2 output, $\dot{V}_A$ is the alveolar ventilation, and K is a constant (see Appendix for a list of symbols). This means that if the alveolar ventilation is halved, the P_{CO_2} is doubled. If the patient does not have a raised arterial P_{CO_2}, he is not hypoventilating!

Second, the hypoxemia can easily be abolished by increasing the inspired P_{O_2} by delivering oxygen via a face mask. this can be seen from the *alveolar gas equation*:

$$P_{A_{O_2}} = P_{I_{O_2}} - \frac{P_{a_{CO_2}}}{R} + F \qquad [2]$$

where F is a small correction factor which we shall ignore. This equation states that if the arterial P_{CO_2} ($P_{a_{CO_2}}$) and respiratory exchange ratio (R) remain constant (they will if the alveolar ventilation and metabolic rate remain unaltered), every mm Hg rise in inspired P_{O_2} ($P_{I_{O_2}}$) will produce a corresponding rise in alveolar P_{O_2} ($P_{a_{O_2}}$). Since it is easily possible to increase the inspired P_{O_2} by several hundred mm Hg, the hypoxemia of pure hypoventilation can be readily abolished.

It is also important to appreciate that the arterial P_{O_2} cannot fall to very low levels from pure hypoventilation. Referring to equation [2] again we can see that if R = 1, the alveolar P_{O_2} falls 1 mm Hg for every 1 mm Hg rise in P_{CO_2}. This means that severe hypoventilation sufficient to double the P_{CO_2} from 40 to 80 mm Hg will only decrease the alveolar P_{O_2} from, say, 100 to 60 mm Hg. Figures 2.3 and 2.4 show that if R = 0.8, the fall is somewhat greater, say, to 50 mm Hg. Also, the arterial P_{O_2} is usually a few mm Hg lower than the alveolar value. But even so, the arterial O_2 saturation will be near 80% and cyanosis will probably be just detectable. However, this is a severe degree of CO_2 retention, which may result in substantial respiratory acidosis, with a pH of around 7.2 and a very sick patient! Thus, hypoxemia is not the dominant feature of hypoventilation.

The causes of hypoventilation are shown in Figure 2.5. They include *1*, depression of the respiratory center by drugs (especially barbiturate and morphine derivatives) or anesthesia; *2*, diseases of the medulla including encephalitis, trauma, hemorrhage, or neoplasm (rare); *3*, abnormalities of the spinal conducting pathways, as following high cervical dislocation; *4*, anterior horn cell diseases such as poliomyelitis; *5*, diseases of the nerves to the respiratory muscles including the Guillain-Barré syndrome and diphtheria; *6*, diseases of the myoneural junction such as myasthenia gravis and anticholinesterase poisoning; *7*, diseases of the respiratory muscles, for example, progressive muscular dystrophy; *8*, thoracic cage abnormalities such as crushed chest;

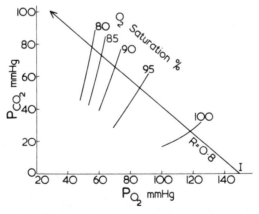

Figure 2.3. O_2–CO_2 diagram showing the relationship between the alveolar P_{O_2} and P_{CO_2} during hypoventilation (respiratory exchange ratio equals 0.8). Note that the P_{CO_2} can rise to approximately 80 mm Hg before the O_2 saturation falls below 80%.

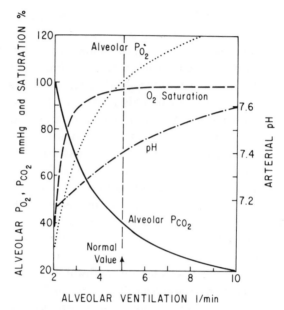

Figure 2.4. Gas exchange during hypoventilation. Values are approximate only.

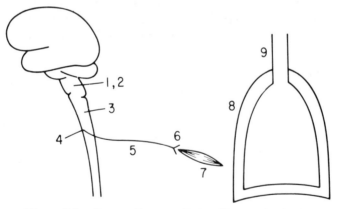

Figure 2.5. Causes of hypoventilation. (See text for details.)

9, upper airway obstruction such as tracheal compression by a thy-
moma or aortic aneurysm.

In addition, hypoventilation is seen in some extremely obese patients
who also have somnolence, polycythemia, and excessive appetite. This
has been dubbed the "pickwickian syndrome" after the fat boy, Joe,

in Charles Dickens's *Pickwick Papers*. The cause of the hypoventilation is uncertain, but the increased work of breathing associated with obesity is probably a factor, though some patients appear to have an abnormality of the central nervous system. There is also a rare condition of idiopathic hypoventilation of unknown cause.

Sleep apnea is a condition which has recently received much attention. It can be divided into *central*, in which there are no respiratory efforts, and *obstructive*, where in spite of activity of the respiratory muscles there is no airflow. *Central sleep apnea* often occurs in patients with hypoventilation because respiratory drive is depressed during sleep. It is known that during REM sleep breathing is often irregular and unresponsive to chemical and vagal drives. An exception is hypoxemia which remains a powerful stimulus to breathe.

Obstructive sleep apnea is much commoner than was once thought. The first reports were in extremely obese patients, but it is now recognized that the condition is not confined to these. Airway obstruction can be caused by backward movement of the tongue, collapse of the pharyngeal walls, or greatly enlarged tonsils or adenoids. Loud snoring often occurs and the patient may wake violently after an apneic episode. There is sometimes chronic sleep deprivation and the patient may have daytime somnolence, chronic fatigue, morning headaches, and often personality disturbances such as paranoia, hostility, and agitated depression.

A condition affecting infants is the *sudden infant death syndrome* (SIDS). Here the child is typically found dead in the cot with no apparent cause. The etiology of this is still obscure. One hypothesis is that the nervous control of ventilation is not fully developed and the respiratory muscles are poorly coordinated.

Diffusion Impairment. This means that equilibration does not occur between the P_{O_2} in the pulmonary capillary blood and alveolar gas. Figure 2.6 reminds us of the time course for P_{O_2} along a pulmonary capillary. Under normal resting conditions, the capillary blood P_{O_2} almost reaches that of alveolar gas after about ⅓ of the total contact time of ¾ sec available in the capillary. Thus, there is plenty of time in reserve. Even on severe exercise when the contact time may be reduced to as little as ¼ sec, equilibration is virtually assured.

In some diseases the blood-gas barrier is thickened and diffusion is so slowed that equilibration may be incomplete. Figure 2.7 shows a

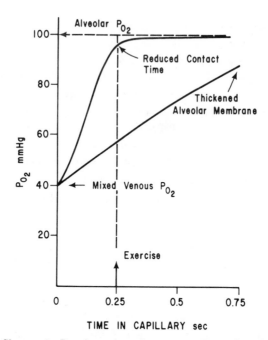

Figure 2.6. Changes in P_{O_2} along the pulmonary capillary. On exercise the time available for O_2 diffusion across the blood-gas barrier is reduced. A thickened alveolar wall slows the rate of diffusion.

histological section of lung from a patient with interstitial fibrosis (5). Note that the normally delicate alveolar walls are grossly widened. In such a lung, we would expect a slower time course as shown in Figure 2.6. Any hypoxemia which occurred at rest would be exaggerated on exercise because of the reduced contact time.

Diseases in which diffusion impairment may contribute to the hypoxemia, especially on exercise, include asbestosis, sarcoidosis, diffuse interstitial fibrosis including the Hamman-Rich syndrome and interstitial pneumonia, collagen diseases affecting the lung including scleroderma, rheumatoid lung, lupus erythematosus, Wegener's granulomatosis, Goodpasture's syndrome, and alveolar cell carcinoma. In all these conditions the diffusion path from alveolar gas to red blood cell may be increased, at least in some regions of the lung, and the time course for oxygenation may be affected, as shown in Figure 2.6.

However, the importance of diffusion impairment to the arterial hypoxemia of these patients is uncertain. As has been emphasized, the

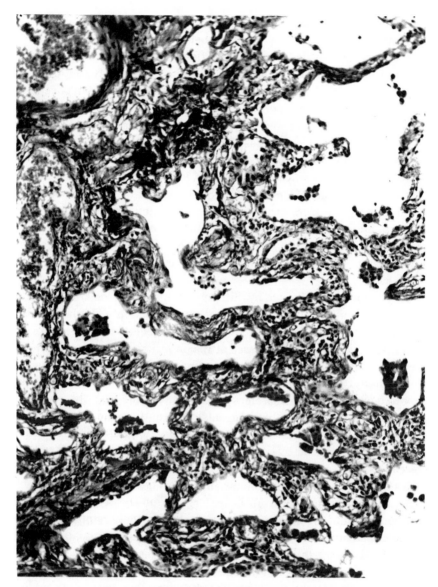

Figure 2.7. Section of lung from a patient with diffuse interstitial fibrosis. Note the marked thickening of the alveolar walls, which constitutes a barrier to diffusion (compare Figures 5.1, 5.3, and 10.5). (From K. F. W. Hinson: Diffuse pulmonary fibrosis. *Hum. Pathol.* 1:275–288, 1970 (5).)

normal lung has lots of diffusion time in reserve. In addition, if we look at Figure 2.7, it is impossible to believe that the normal relationships between ventilation and blood flow can be preserved in a lung with such an abnormal architecture. We shall see shortly that uneven ventilation-perfusion relationships are a powerful cause of hypoxemia, which is undoubtedly operating in these patients. Thus, how much additional hypoxemia should be attributed to diffusion impairment is difficult to know. Recent measurements suggest that at least some of the hypoxemia on exercise is caused by this mechanism (Figure 5.6).

Another possible way in which hypoxemia could result would be an extreme reduction in contact time. Suppose that so much blood flow is diverted away from other regions of the lung (for example, by a large pulmonary embolus) that the time for oxygenation within the capillary is reduced to $\frac{1}{10}$th normal. Figure 2.6 shows that hypoxemia would then be inevitable. Whether this ever occurs in practice is unknown.

Any hypoxemia caused by diffusion impairment can be readily corrected by administering 100% oxygen to the patient. This is because the resultant large increase in alveolar P_{O_2} of several hundred mm Hg can easily overcome the increased diffusion resistance of the thickened alveolar membrane. Carbon dioxide elimination is generally thought to be unaffected by diffusion abnormalities, although recent work has raised questions about this. Certainly most patients with the diseases listed above do not have carbon dioxide retention. Indeed, typically the arterial P_{CO_2} is slightly lower than normal because ventilation is overstimulated, either by the hypoxemia or by intrapulmonary stretch receptors.

Shunt. This means that some blood reaches the arterial system without passing through ventilated regions of the lung. The most common shunts are extrapulmonary, including those which occur in congenital heart disease through atrial or ventricular septal defects or a patent ductus arteriosus. In such patients there must be a rise in right heart pressure; otherwise the shunt is from left to right. Intrapulmonary shunts can be caused by arterial-venous fistulas. In addition, a completely unventilated but perfused area of lung, for example, a consolidated pneumonic lobule, constitutes a shunt. It might be argued that the latter is simply one extreme of the spectrum of ventilation-perfusion ratios and that therefore it is more reasonable to classify hypoxemia caused by this under the heading of ventilation-perfusion inequality, but a shunt causes such a characteristic pattern of gas exchange during 100% oxygen breathing that it is convenient to include unventilated alveoli under this heading.

If a patient with a shunt is given pure oxygen to breathe, the arterial P_{O_2} fails to rise to the level seen in normal subjects. Figure 2.8 reminds us of the reason for this. While the end-capillary P_{O_2} may be as high as that in alveolar gas, the P_{O_2} and the O_2 content of the shunted blood are as low as in venous blood. A mixture of the two bloods therefore causes a large fall in P_{O_2} because the O_2 dissociation curve is so flat in its upper range. As a result, it is possible to detect small shunts by measuring the arterial P_{O_2} during 100% O_2 breathing.

Only shunts behave in this way, a point of great practical importance. In the other three causes of hypoxemia—hypoventilation, diffusion impairment, and ventilation-perfusion inequality—the arterial P_{O_2} nearly reaches the level seen in normal subjects during 100% O_2 breathing. However, this may take a very long time in some patients with very poorly ventilated alveoli because the nitrogen takes so long to wash out completely that the P_{O_2} is slow to reach its final level. This is apparently the reason why the arterial P_{O_2} of patients with

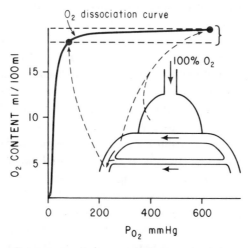

Figure 2.8. Shunt during 100% O_2 breathing. The addition of a small amount of shunted blood with its low O_2 content greatly reduces the P_{O_2} of arterial blood. This is because the O_2 dissociation curve is so flat when the P_{O_2} is very high.

chronic obstructive lung disease may only rise to 400–500 mm Hg after 15 min of 100% O_2 breathing.

The magnitude of the shunt during O_2 breathing can be determined from the *shunt equation*:

$$\frac{\dot{Q}_S}{\dot{Q}_T} = \frac{C_{c'} - C_a}{C_{c'} - C_{\bar{v}}}$$ [3]

where $\dot{Q}_S$ and $\dot{Q}_T$ refer to the shunt and total blood flows, and $C_{c}{}'$, C_a and $C_{\bar{v}}$ refer to the O_2 contents of end-capillary, arterial, and mixed venous blood. The O_2 content of end-capillary blood is calculated from the alveolar P_{O_2} assuming complete equilibration between the alveolar gas and the blood. Mixed venous blood is sampled with a catheter in the pulmonary artery. Alternatively the denominator in equation [3] can be calculated from the measured oxygen uptake and cardiac output. Sometimes a figure of 5 ml/100 ml is assumed but this can lead to substantial errors.

Shunt does not usually result in a raised arterial P_{CO_2}. The tendency for this to rise is generally countered by the chemoreceptors which increase ventilation if the P_{CO_2} increases. Indeed, often the arterial P_{CO_2} is lower than normal because of the additional hypoxemic stimulus to ventilation.

Ventilation-Perfusion Inequality. This means that ventilation and blood flow are mismatched in various regions of the lung, with the result that all gas transfer becomes inefficient. This mechanism of hypoxemia is extremely common; it is responsible for most if not all of the hypoxemia of chronic obstructive lung disease, interstitial lung disease, and vascular disorders such as pulmonary embolism. It is generally identified by excluding the other three causes of hypoxemia: hypoventilation, diffusion impairment, and shunt.

All lungs have some ventilation-perfusion inequality. In the normal upright lung this takes the form of a regional pattern, with the ventilation-perfusion ratio decreasing from apex to base. But as disease occurs and progresses we see a disorganization of this pattern until eventually the normal relationships between ventilation and blood flow are destroyed at the alveolar level. (For a discussion of the physiology of how ventilation-perfusion inequality causes hypoxemia, the reader is referred to the companion volume, J. B. West: *Respiratory Physiology—The Essentials*, ed. 3, pp. 57–66.)

Several factors can exaggerate the hypoxemia of ventilation-perfusion inequality. One is concomitant hypoventilation, which may occur if a patient with severe chronic obstructive lung disease is sedated. Another factor which is frequently overlooked is a reduction in cardiac output. This causes a fall of P_{O_2} in mixed venous blood, which results in a fall of arterial P_{O_2} for the same degree of ventilation-perfusion inequality. This situation is often seen in patients who develop a myocardial infarct with mild pulmonary edema.

How can we assess the severity of ventilation-perfusion inequality from the arterial blood gases? First, the *arterial* P_{O_2} is a useful guide. A patient with an arterial P_{O_2} of 40 mm Hg is very likely to have more ventilation-perfusion inequality than a patient with an arterial P_{O_2} of 70 mm Hg. But we can be misled. For example, suppose that the first patient had reduced his ventilation, with the result that the alveolar P_{O_2} had fallen by 30 mm Hg, thus pulling down the arterial P_{O_2}. Under these conditions, the arterial P_{O_2} by itself would be deceptive. For this reason, we often calculate the *alveolar-arterial difference* for P_{O_2}.

What should we use for alveolar P_{O_2}? Figure 2.9 reminds us that in a lung with ventilation-perfusion inequality, there may be a wide spectrum of values for alveolar P_{O_2}, ranging from inspired gas to mixed venous blood. Riley and Cournand (6) suggested that we calculate an

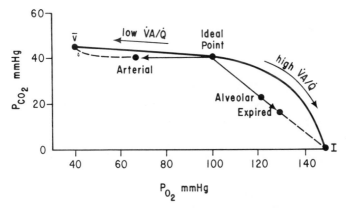

Figure 2.9. O_2–CO_2 diagram showing the arterial, ideal, alveolar, and expired points. The *curved line* indicates the P_{O_2} and P_{CO_2} of all lung units having different ventilation-perfusion ratios.*

* For additional information on this difficult topic, see J. B. West: *Respiratory Physiology—The Essentials*, ed. 3, pp. 57 and 151. Baltimore, Williams & Wilkins, 1985.

"ideal alveolar P_{O_2}." This is the value that the lung *would* have if there were no ventilation-perfusion inequality and the respiratory exchange ratio remained the same. It is found from the alveolar gas equation:

$$P_{A_{O_2}} = P_{I_{O_2}} - \frac{P_{a_{CO_2}}}{R} + F$$

using the respiratory exchange ratio R of the whole lung, and assuming that arterial and alveolar P_{CO_2} are the same (usually they nearly are). Thus, the *alveolar-arterial difference* for P_{O_2} makes an allowance for the effect of any under- or over-ventilation on the arterial P_{O_2} and is a purer measure of ventilation-perfusion inequality.

But even this index can be misleading because of the shape of the O_2 dissociation curve. An alveolar-arterial P_{O_2} difference of 30 mm Hg high on the dissociation curve when the alveolar P_{O_2} is 120 and the arterial P_{O_2} is 90 because of an increased ventilation indicates less disease than the same P_{O_2} difference lower on the curve when the alveolar P_{O_2} is 100. For this reason the *physiological shunt* is often calculated. This is the amount of venous blood which would have to be mixed with "ideal" blood to give the observed arterial P_{O_2}. We know that true shunting of blood is not responsible for the hypoxemia, but nevertheless it is useful to calculate this "as if" value. This is done with the shunt equation in the form:

$$\frac{\dot{Q}_{PS}}{\dot{Q}_T} = \frac{C_i - C_a}{C_i - C_{\bar{v}}} \qquad [4]$$

where $\dot{Q}_{PS}$ is the physiological shunt and Ci is the O_2 content of ideal end-capillary blood. This index is less sensitive to the levels of overall ventilation and blood flow. The normal value is less than 5%. In patients with acute respiratory failure it may rise to over 50%.

The physiological shunt is chiefly caused by lung units with low ventilation-perfusion ratios which lie to the left of the ideal point on Figure 2.9 and "pull" the arterial point to the left. To get information about alveoli with high ventilation-perfusion ratios, the *physiological dead space* is calculated. To do this, we pretend that all the movement of the expired point from the ideal point is caused by the addition of dead space gas, including the anatomical dead space. The equation is

$$\frac{V_D}{V_T} = \frac{P_i - P_E}{P_i} \qquad [5]$$

where $\dfrac{V_D}{V_T}$ is the dead space to tidal volume ratio and P_i and P_E refer

to the P_{CO_2} in ideal and mixed expired gas. Since the P_{CO_2} in ideal gas and arterial blood are virtually the same (Figure 2.9), we can use the equation

$$\frac{V_D}{V_T} = \frac{P_a - P_E}{P_a}$$

where P_a is the arterial P_{CO_2}.

The normal value for physiological dead space is about 30% of the tidal volume at rest and less on exercise, and it consists almost completely of anatomical dead space. In chronic lung disease it may rise to 50% or more due to the presence of ventilation-perfusion inequality.

It is possible to obtain more information about the distribution of ventilation-perfusion ratios in the lung with a technique based on the elimination of injected foreign gases (7). A series of six inert gases dissolved in saline is slowly infused into a peripheral vein, and after a steady state of elimination by the lung has been achieved, the concentrations are measured in the arterial blood and expired gas by gas chromatography. Because the gases have different solubilities, they partition themselves between blood and gas according to the ventilation-perfusion ratio of the lung unit. It is thus possible to derive a virtually continuous distribution of ventilation-perfusion ratios which is consistent with the measured pattern of elimination of the six gases. Figure 2.10 shows a typical pattern found in young normal volunteers; it can be seen that almost all the ventilation and blood flow go to lung units with ventilation-perfusion ratios near the normal value of 1. As we shall see subsequently, this pattern is greatly disturbed by lung disease.

Mixed Causes of Hypoxemia. These frequently occur. For example, a patient who is being ventilated because of acute respiratory failure following an automobile accident may have a large shunt through unventilated lung in addition to severe ventilation-perfusion inequality (Figure 8.3). Again, a patient with interstitial lung disease may have some diffusion impairment, but this will certainly be accompanied by ventilation-perfusion inequality and possibly by shunt as well (Figure 5.6). In our present state of knowledge it is often impossible to

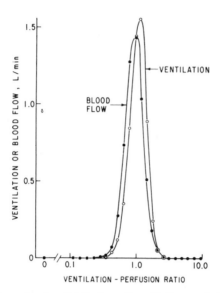

Figure 2.10. Example of a distribution of ventilation-perfusion ratios in a young normal subject as obtained by the multiple inert gas elimination technique. Note that most of the ventilation and blood flow go to lung units with ventilation-perfusion ratios near 1. (From P. D. Wagner, R. B. Laravuso, R. R. Uhl, and J. B. West: Continuous distributions of ventilation-perfusion ratios in normal subjects breathing air and 100% O_2. *J. Clin. Invest.* 54:54–68, 1974 (7).)

accurately define the mechanism of hypoxemia, especially in the acutely ill patient.

Oxygen Delivery. Although the P_{O_2} of arterial blood is of great importance, other factors enter into the delivery of oxygen to the tissues. For example, a reduced arterial P_{O_2} in a patient with a hemoglobin of 5 g/100 ml is clearly more detrimental than in a patient with a normal O_2 capacity. The delivery of oxygen to the tissues depends on the oxygen capacity of the blood, the cardiac output, and the distribution of blood flow to the periphery. These factors are discussed further on page 177.

Arterial P_{CO_2}

Measurement

A P_{CO_2} electrode as shown in Figure 2.1 is used. This is essentially a glass pH electrode surrounded by a bicarbonate buffer, which is separated from the blood by a thin membrane through which CO_2

diffuses. The CO_2 alters the pH of the buffer, and this is measured by the electrode which reads out the P_{CO_2} directly. Calibration is by means of gas with a known P_{CO_2}.

Normal Values

The normal arterial P_{CO_2} is 37–43 mm Hg and is unaffected by age. It tends to fall slightly on heavy exercise and to rise slightly during sleep. Sometimes a blood sample obtained by arterial puncture will show a value in the low 30's. This can be attributed to the acute hyperventilation caused by the procedure and can be recognized by the correspondingly increased pH.

Causes of Increased Arterial P_{CO_2}

There are two major causes of CO_2 retention:

1. Hypoventilation
2. Ventilation-perfusion inequality

Hypoventilation. This was dealt with in some detail above, where we saw that hypoventilation must cause hypoxemia and CO_2 retention, the latter being more important (Figures 2.3 and 2.4). The *alveolar ventilation equation*

$$P_{A_{CO_2}} = \frac{\dot{V}_{CO_2}}{\dot{V}_A} \cdot K$$

emphasizes the inverse relationship between the ventilation and the alveolar P_{CO_2}. In normal lungs the arterial P_{CO_2} closely follows the alveolar value. Whereas the hypoxemia of hypoventilation can be easily relieved by increasing the inspired P_{O_2}, the CO_2 retention can only be treated by increasing the ventilation. This may require mechanical assistance, as described in Chapter 10.

Ventilation-Perfusion Inequality. Although this was considered above, its relationship to CO_2 retention warrants further brief discussion because of confusion in this area. At one time it was argued that ventilation-perfusion inequality does not interfere with CO_2 elimination because the overventilated regions make up for the underventilated areas. This is a fallacy, and it is important to realize that ventilation-perfusion inequality reduces the efficiency of transfer of all gases, including, for example, the anesthetic gases.

Why then do we frequently see patients with chronic lung disease and undoubted ventilation-perfusion inequality who have a normal arterial P_{CO_2}? Figure 2.11 shows the usual sequence. The normal relationships between ventilation and blood flow (A) are disturbed by disease, and hypoxemia and CO_2 retention develop (B). But the chemoreceptors respond to the increased arterial P_{CO_2} and raise the ventilation to the alveoli. The result is that the arterial P_{CO_2} is returned to its normal level (C). However, although the arterial P_{O_2} is somewhat raised by the increased ventilation, it does not return all the way to normal. This can be explained by the shape of the O_2 dissociation curve and in particular the strongly depressive action on the arterial P_{O_2} of lung units with low ventilation-perfusion ratios. Whereas units with high ventilation-perfusion ratios are very effective at eliminating CO_2, they have little advantage over normal units in taking up O_2. The end result is that the arterial P_{CO_2} is effectively lowered to the normal value, but there is relatively little rise in arterial P_{O_2}.

Some patients do not make the transition from stage B to C, or having made it, revert to B and develop CO_2 retention. What is the reason for this? Generally these patients have a very high work of breathing, often because of a gross increase in airway resistance. Apparently they elect to raise their P_{CO_2} rather than to expend the extra energy to increase ventilation. It is of interest that if normal subjects are made to breathe through a narrow tube, thus increasing their work of breathing, their alveolar P_{CO_2} often rises.

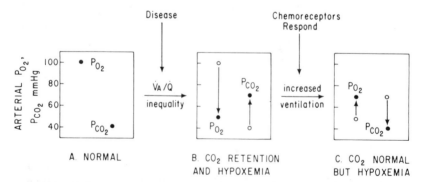

Figure 2.11. Arterial P_{O_2} and P_{CO_2} in different stages of ventilation-perfusion inequality. Initially there must be both a fall in P_{O_2} and a rise in P_{CO_2}. However, when the ventilation to the alveoli is increased, the P_{CO_2} returns to normal but the P_{O_2} remains abnormally low.

We do not fully understand why some patients with ventilation-perfusion inequality increase their ventilation and some do not. As we shall see in Chapter 5, many patients with emphysema hold their P_{CO_2} at the normal level even when their disease is far advanced. Patients with asthma generally do the same. This can involve a very large increase in ventilation to their alveoli. On the other hand, other patients, for example, those with severe chronic bronchitis, typically allow their P_{CO_2} to rise much earlier in the course of the disease. It is possible that there is some difference in the central neurogenic control of ventilation in these two groups of patients.

Arterial pH

Measurement

This is usually measured with a glass electrode concurrently with the arterial P_{O_2} and P_{CO_2}. The acid-base status of the blood is closely linked to the arterial P_{CO_2} through the Henderson-Hasselbalch equation:

$$pH = pK + \log \frac{(HCO_3^-)}{0.03 \ P_{CO_2}}$$

where $pK = 6.1$ and (HCO_3^-) is the plasma bicarbonate concentration in milliequivalents per liter.

Acidosis

This means a decrease in arterial pH or a process which tends to do this. Sometimes the term "acidemia" is used to refer to the actual fall in pH. Acidosis can be caused by respiratory or metabolic abnormalities, or (frequently) both.

Respiratory Acidosis. This is caused by CO_2 retention, which increases the denominator in the Henderson-Hasselbalch equation and so depresses the pH. We have seen that there are two mechanisms of CO_2 retention: hypoventilation and ventilation-perfusion ratio inequality. Both can cause respiratory acidosis.

It is important to distinguish between acute and chronic CO_2 retention. A patient with hypoventilation following an overdose of barbiturate is likely to develop acute respiratory acidosis. There is little change in bicarbonate concentration (the numerator in the Henderson-Hasselbalch equation), and the pH therefore falls rapidly as the

P_{CO_2} rises. Typically, a doubling of the P_{CO_2} from 40 to 80 mm Hg in such a patient reduces the pH from 7.4 to about 7.2.

By contrast, a patient who develops chronic CO_2 retention over a period of many weeks as a result of increasing ventilation-perfusion inequality caused by chronic lung disease typically has a smaller fall in pH. This is because the kidneys retain bicarbonate in response to the increased P_{CO_2} in the renal tubular cells, increasing the numerator in the Henderson-Hasselbalch equation (partially compensated respiratory acidosis).

These relationships are shown diagrammatically in Figure 2.12 (8). Contrast the steep slope of the line for acute CO_2 retention (A) with the shallow slope of the line for chronic hypercapnia (B). Note also that a patient with acute hypoventilation whose P_{CO_2} is maintained over 2 or 3 days will move toward the chronic line as his kidney conserves bicarbonate (point A to C). Conversely, a patient with chronic obstructive lung disease with long-standing CO_2 retention who develops an acute chest infection with worsening of his ventilation-

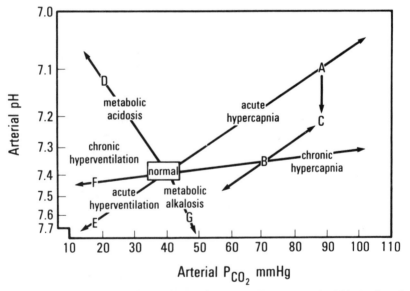

Figure 2.12. Arterial pH-P_{CO_2} relationships in various types of acid-base disturbances. (See text for details.) (Modified from D. C. Flenley: Another non-logarithmic acid-base diagram? *Lancet* 1:961–965, 1971 (8).)

perfusion relationships may move rapidly from point B to C, that is, parallel to line A. On the other hand, if he is then artificially ventilated, he may move back to point B, or even beyond.

Metabolic Acidosis.   This is caused by a primary fall in the numerator (HCO_3^-) of the Henderson-Hasselbalch equation, an example being uncontrolled diabetes mellitus. Uncompensated metabolic acidosis would be indicated by a vertical upward movement on Figure 2.12, but in practice the fall in arterial pH stimulates the peripheral chemoreceptors, increasing the ventilation and lowering the P_{CO_2}. As a result, the pH and P_{CO_2} move along line D.

Lactic acidosis is another form of metabolic acidosis, and this may complicate severe acute respiratory failure as a consequence of tissue hypoxia. If such a patient is artificially ventilated, the pH will remain below 7.4 when the P_{CO_2} is returned to normal.

Alkalosis (or Alkalemia)

This means an increase in arterial pH.

Respiratory Alkalosis.   This is seen in acute hysterical hyperventilation where the pH rises, as in E in Figure 2.12. If the hyperventilation is maintained, for example, at high altitude, compensated respiratory alkalosis is seen, with a return of the pH toward normal as the kidney excretes bicarbonate, a movement from E to F.

Metabolic Alkalosis.   This is seen in severe prolonged vomiting, when the plasma bicarbonate concentration rises, as in G in Figure 2.12. The arterial P_{CO_2} typically increases a little because of slight respiratory depression though sometimes no change occurs. Metabolic alkalosis also occurs when a patient with long-standing lung disease and compensated respiratory acidosis is ventilated too enthusiastically, thus bringing his P_{CO_2} rapidly to nearly 40 mm Hg (line B to G). Another form is seen when potassium chloride deficiency occurs in a patient whose ventilatory failure is successfully treated.

DIFFUSING CAPACITY

So far this chapter on gas exchange has been devoted to arterial blood gases and their significance. However, this is a convenient place to discuss another common test of gas exchange, the diffusing capacity of the lung for carbon monoxide.

Measurement of Diffusing Capacity

This most popular method of measuring the diffusing capacity (D_{CO}) is the single breath method (Figure 2.13). The patient takes a vital capacity breath of 0.3% CO and 10% helium, holds his breath for 10 sec, and then exhales. The first 750 ml of gas are discarded because of dead space contamination and the next liter is collected and analyzed. The helium gives the dilution of the inspired gas with alveolar gas and thus the initial alveolar P_{CO}. On the assumption that the CO is lost from alveolar gas in proportion to the P_{CO} during breathholding, the diffusing capacity is calculated as the volume of CO taken up per minute per mm Hg alveolar P_{CO}. The diffusing capacity can also be measured by inhaling CO at a low concentration during normal breathing, the so-called steady-state method.

Causes of Reduced Diffusing Capacity

CO is used to measure diffusing capacity because when it is inhaled in low concentrations, the partial pressure in the pulmonary capillary blood remains extremely low in relation to the alveolar value. As a result, CO is taken up by the blood all along the capillary (contrast

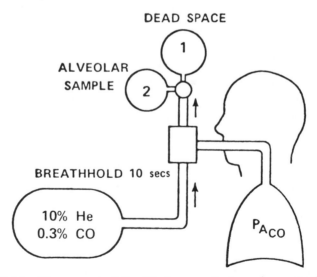

Figure 2.13. Measurement of the diffusing capacity for carbon monoxide by the single breath method. The subject takes a single breath of 0.3% CO with 10% helium, holds his breath for 10 sec, and then exhales. After discarding of the first 750 ml, an alveolar sample is collected and analyzed.

the time course of O_2 shown in Figure 2.6). Thus, the uptake of CO is determined by the *diffusion properties* of the blood-gas barrier and the *rate of combination* of CO with blood.

The *diffusion properties* of the alveolar membrane depend on its thickness and area. Thus, the diffusing capacity is reduced by diseases in which the thickness is increased, including diffuse interstitial fibrosis, sarcoidosis, and asbestosis (Figure 2.7). It is also reduced when the area of the blood-gas barrier is reduced, for example, by pneumonectomy. The fall in diffusing capacity which occurs in emphysema may be caused by the loss of alveolar walls and capillaries (but see below).

The *rate of combination* of CO with blood is reduced whenever the number of red cells in the capillaries is reduced. This occurs in anemia and also diseases which reduce the capillary blood volume, such as pulmonary embolism. It is possible to separate the membrane and blood components of the diffusing capacity by making the measurement at a high and normal alveolar P_{O_2}.

Interpretation of Diffusing Capacity

Unfortunately, in many patients in whom the measured diffusing capacity is low, the interpretation is uncertain. The reason for this is the unevenness of ventilation, bloodflow, and diffusion properties throughout the diseased lung. We know that such lungs tend to empty unevenly (Figure 1.11), so that the liter of expired gas which is analyzed for CO (Figure 2.13) is probably not representative of the whole lung. A reflection of this problem is that different methods of measuring diffusing capacity in patients with diseased lungs frequently show poor agreement.

For this reason, the diffusing capacity is sometimes referred to as the transfer factor (especially in Europe) to emphasize that it is more a measure of the lung's overall ability to transfer gas into the blood than a specific test of diffusion characteristics. However, in spite of this uncertainty of interpretation, the test has a definite place in the pulmonary function laboratory and is frequently useful in assessing the severity and type of lung disease.

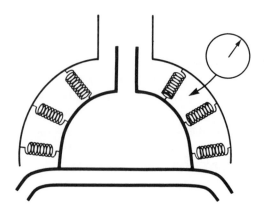

chapter 3

Other Tests

In the first two chapters, we concentrated on two simple but very informative tests of pulmonary function: the forced expiration, and arterial blood gases. In this chapter we shall briefly consider some of the other ways of measuring lung function. Of the large number of possible tests which have been introduced from time to time, only the most useful will be selected, and the principles rather than the details of their use will be emphasized.

STATIC LUNG VOLUMES

Measurement

The measurement of the vital capacity with a simple spirometer was described in Chapter 1 (Figure 1.1). This equipment can also be used to obtain the tidal volume, inspiratory capacity, and expiratory reserve volume (functional residual capacity minus the residual volume). However, the residual volume, functional residual capacity, and total lung capacity require additional measurements.

The *functional residual capacity* (FRC) can be measured with a body plethysmograph, which is essentially a large airtight box in which the

42

patient sits.* The mouthpiece is obstructed, and the patient is instructed to make rapid panting efforts. As he compresses the gas volume in his lungs, the air in the plethysmograph expands slightly and its pressure falls. By applying Boyle's law, the lung volume can be obtained. Another method is to use the helium dilution technique, in which a spirometer of known volume and helium concentration is connected to the patient in a closed circuit. From the degree of dilution of the helium, the unknown lung volume can be calculated. The *residual volume* (RV) can be derived from the FRC by subtracting the expiratory reserve volume.

Interpretation

The FRC and RV often are increased in diseases in which there is an increased airway resistance, for example, emphysema, chronic bronchitis, and asthma. Indeed, at one time an elevated RV was regarded as an essential feature of emphysema, but less emphasis is placed on this test now. The RV is raised in these conditions chiefly because airway closure occurs at an abnormally high lung volume.

A reduced FRC and RV are often seen in patients with reduced lung compliance, for example, in diffuse interstitial fibrosis. Here the lung is stiff and tends to recoil to a smaller resting volume.

If the FRC is measured by both the plethysmographic and gas dilution methods, a comparison of the two results is often informative. The plethysmographic method measures all the gas in the lung. However, the dilution techniques only "see" those regions of lung which communicate with the mouth. Therefore, regions behind closed airways, for example, cysts, will result in a higher value for the plethysmographic than for the dilution procedures. The same disparity is often seen in patients with chronic obstructive lung disease, probably because some areas are so poorly ventilated that they do not equilibrate in the time allowed.

LUNG ELASTICITY

Measurement

The pressure-volume curve of the lung requires knowledge of the pressures both in the airways and around the lung. A good estimate of

---

* See J. B. West: *Respiratory Physiology—The Essentials*, ed. 3, p. 14. Baltimore, Williams & Wilkins, 1985.

the latter can be obtained from the esophageal pressure. A small balloon on the end of a catheter is passed down through the nose or mouth, and the difference between the mouth and esophageal pressures is recorded as the patient exhales in steps of 1 liter from total lung capacity (TLC) to RV. The resulting pressure-volume curve is not linear (Figure 3.1), so that a single value for its slope (compliance) is often misleading. However, the compliance is sometimes reported for the liter above FRC measured on the descending limb of the pressure-volume curve.

The pressure-volume curve is often reported using the percentage of predicted TLC on the vertical axis rather than the actual lung volume in liters (Figure 3.1) (9). This procedure helps to allow for differences in body size and reduces the variability of the results. Normal values for compliance are given in the Appendix.

Interpretation

Elastic recoil is reduced in patients with emphysema. Figure 3.1 shows that the pressure-volume curve is displaced to the left and has a steeper slope in this condition, presumably as a result of the destruction of the alveolar walls (Figures 4.2, 4.3, and 4.5) and the consequent disorganization of elastic tissue. The change in compliance is not reversible. The pressure-volume curve is also typically shifted to the

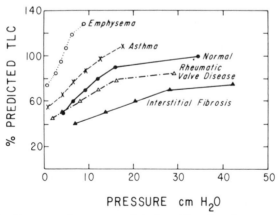

Figure 3.1.   Pressure-volume curves of the lung. Note that the curves for emphysema and asthma (during bronchospasm) are shifted upward and to the left while those for rheumatic valve disease and interstitial fibrosis are flattened. (From D. V. Bates, P. T. Macklem, and R. V. Christie: *Respiratory Function in Disease*, ed. 2. Philadelphia, W. B. Saunders, 1971 (9).)

left in patients with asthma during an attack, but the change is reversible in some patients. The reasons for this shift are obscure. Increasing age also tends to reduce elastic recoil.

Elastic recoil is increased in interstitial lung disease, which results in the deposition of fibrous tissue in the alveolar walls (Figures 2.7 and 5.3), reducing their distensibility. Elastic recoil also tends to increase in patients with rheumatic heart disease who have a raised pulmonary capillary pressure and some interstitial edema. However, it should be noted that measurements of the pressure-volume curve show considerable variability and the neat results shown in Figure 3.1 are based on the means of many patients.

AIRWAY RESISTANCE

Measurement

This is defined as the pressure difference between the alveoli and the mouth divided by the flow rate. Alveolar pressure can only be measured indirectly: one way to do this is with a body plethysmograph.* The subject sits inside the airtight box and pants through a flowmeter. The alveolar pressure can be deduced from the pressure changes in the plethysmograph because, when the alveolar gas is compressed, the plethysmograph gas volume increases slightly, causing a fall in pressure. This method has the great advantage that lung volume can be easily measured almost simultaneously. Figure 3.2 shows the effect of cigarette smoking on airway resistance, here expressed as its reciprocal, conductance (10).

Other methods of measuring airway resistance are in use. In one, lung volume, flow rate, and esophageal pressure are measured simultaneously; airway resistance is derived by subtracting the pressure component responsible for the change in lung volume.† This method has the disadvantage that an esophageal catheter is necessary, but it allows lung compliance to be measured at the same time. Since tissue resistance is included in this measurement, the result is often called *pulmonary resistance.* Another method is to connect the subject to a source of forced air oscillations, such as a loudspeaker, and measure the relationship between pressure and flow at the mouth. Finally, an

* See J. B. West: *Respiratory Physiology—The Essentials*, ed. 3, p. 156. Baltimore, Williams & Wilkins, 1985.
† See J. B. West: *Respiratory Physiology—The Essentials*, ed. 3, p. 157. Baltimore, Williams & Wilkins, 1985.

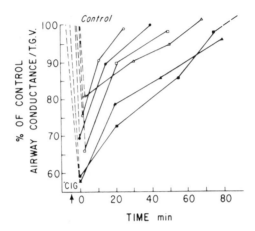

Figure 3.2. Effect of cigarette smoking on airway conductance as measured in the body plethysmograph. The ordinate shows conductance over thoracic gas volume. (From J. A. Nadel and J. H. Comroe, Jr.: Acute effects of inhalation of cigarette smoke on airway conductance. *J. Appl. Physiol.* 16:713–716, 1961 (10).)

interrupter technique is available. In this the airflow is interrupted by a shutter in the mouthpiece 10 times/sec, giving an estimate of alveolar pressure. In general, all these methods are satisfactory in nearly normal lungs, but the interpretation of the results becomes increasingly questionable in the presence of advanced lung disease.

Interpretation

Airway resistance varies inversely with lung volume because the expanding parenchyma exerts traction on the airway walls. Thus, any measurement of airways resistance must be related to the lung volume. It should also be emphasized that the small peripheral airways normally contribute little to overall resistance because there are so many arranged in parallel. For this reason, special tests have been devised to detect early changes in small airways. These include the flow rate during the latter part of the flow-volume curve (Figure 1.8), the flow-volume curve during helium breathing (page 12), closing volume (Figure 1.10), and frequency dependence of compliance.* The last is determined by measuring lung dynamic compliance at frequencies of 10–120 breaths/min. The fall in dynamic compliance with increasing

---

* See J. B. West: *Respiratory Physiology—The Essentials*, ed. 3, p. 150. Baltimore, Williams & Wilkins, 1985.

frequency is due to the uneven time constants caused by diseased peripheral airways. The usefulness of these tests in detecting early disease of the small airways is still being evaluated.

Airway resistance is increased in chronic bronchitis and emphysema. In chronic bronchitis, the lumen of a typical airway contains excessive secretions, and the wall is thickened by mucous gland hyperplasia and edema (Figure 4.6). In emphysema, many of the airways lose their support because of destruction of the alveolar walls that surround them (Figures 4.1 and 4.2). As a result, their resistance may not be increased much during quiet breathing but, with any exertion, dynamic compression (Figure 1.6) quickly occurs on expiration and resistance rises strikingly. Such patients often show a reasonably high flow rate very early in expiration, but this abruptly drops to low values as flow limitation occurs (see the flow-volume curve in Figure 1.8). Recall that the driving pressure under these conditions is the static recoil pressure of the lung (Figure 1.6), which is reduced in emphysema (Figure 3.1).

Airway resistance is also increased in patients with bronchial asthma. Here the factors include contraction of bronchial smooth muscle with resultant bronchoconstriction, mucous plugs occluding many of the airways, and edema of their walls (Figure 4.13). The resistance may be very high during attacks, especially in relation to lung volume, which is frequently much increased. The resistance is reduced by bronchodilator drugs. Even during periods of remission when the patient is asymptomatic, airway resistance may be raised.

Tracheal obstruction causes an increased airway resistance. This may be caused by compression from outside, for example, an enlarged thyroid, or by intrinsic narrowing caused by scarring or a tumor. An important feature is that the obstruction is usually apparent during inspiration and it can be detected on an inspiratory flow-volume curve. In addition, an audible stridor is often present.

INEQUALITY OF VENTILATION

Measurement

Ventilatory inequality can be assessed by the single breath N_2 test, which was discussed on page 14 (Figure 1.10). Another method of measuring the unevenness of ventilation is with a multibreath N_2 washout. The patient is connected to a source of pure O_2 via a valve box, and a rapidly responding N_2 meter records the end-expiratory value of each breath. A uniformly ventilated lung (such as is seen in young normal subjects) will show an exponential fall in end-expiratory N_2 with time because each successive breath washes out the same fraction of the gas left in the lung.* Such a record gives a straight line when N_2 concentration is plotted against breath number (or time) on semilogarithmic paper. However, a diseased lung produces a curved line, because first well-ventilated regions wash out their N_2 rapidly, followed by poorly ventilated regions which wash out their N_2 slowly. Various indices of the abnormal washout pattern have been described.

Interpretation

The interpretation of tests of uneven ventilation was discussed on page 15.

CONTROL OF VENTILATION

Measurement

The ventilatory response to carbon dioxide can be conveniently studied by means of a rebreathing technique (11). A small bag is filled with a mixture of 6–7% CO_2 in oxygen and the patient rebreathes from this over a period of several minutes. The bag P_{CO_2} increases at the rate of 4–6 mm Hg/min, and thus the change in ventilation per mm Hg increase in P_{CO_2} can easily be determined.

The ventilatory response to hypoxia can be measured in a similar way. In this instance the bag is filled with 24% O_2, 7% CO_2, and the balance N_2. During rebreathing, the P_{CO_2} is monitored and held constant by means of a variable bypass and CO_2 absorber. Rebreathing can be continued until the inspired P_{O_2} falls to about 40 mm Hg. This method is technically more difficult than that for the carbon dioxide response and therefore it is less often used.

Both these techniques give information about the overall ventilatory response to CO_2 or hypoxia, but they do not differentiate between patients who will not breathe because of central nervous system or neuromuscular inadequacy on the one hand, and those who cannot breathe because of mechanical abnormalities of the chest on the other. To make this distinction between those who "won't" and those who "can't" breathe, the mechanical work performed during inspiration

* See J. B. West: *Respiratory Physiology—The Essentials*, ed. 3, p. 110. Baltimore, Williams & Wilkins, 1985.

can be measured. To accomplish this the esophageal pressure is recorded together with tidal volume, and the area of the pressure-volume loop is obtained.* Inspiratory work recorded in this way is one useful measure of the neural output of the respiratory center.

Another method of assessing the output of the respiratory center is to measure the inspiratory pressure during a brief period of airway occlusion (12). The patient breathes through a mouthpiece into a valve box which separates the inspired and expired flows, and the inspiratory port is provided with a shutter. This is closed during an expiration (the patient being unaware), so that the first part of his next inspiration is against an occluded airway. The shutter is opened after about ½ sec. However, the pressure generated during the first 0.1 sec of attempted inspiration ($P_{0.1}$) is taken as a measure of respiratory center output. This is largely unaffected by the mechanical properties of the respiratory system, although it may be influenced by lung volume.

Interpretation

The ventilatory response to CO_2 is depressed by sleep, narcotic drugs, and genetic, racial, and personality factors. An important question is why some patients with chronic lung disease develop CO_2 retention and others do not. In this context there are considerable differences of CO_2 response between individuals, and it has been suggested that the course of patients with chronic respiratory disease may be related to this. Thus, patients who respond strongly to a rise in P_{CO2} may be more distressed by dyspnea, while those who respond weakly may succumb to respiratory failure.

Figure 3.3A shows the results in three patients with chronic obstructive lung disease who performed an abnormally small amount of inspiratory work in response to inspired CO_2. In addition they required an inordinately high inspiratory work for a given amount of ventilation (B). Thus, these patients had evidence of both a reduced respiratory center output and mechanical obstruction to breathing (13).

The factors which affect the ventilatory response to hypoxia are less well understood. However, the response is considerably blunted in persons who have been hypoxemic since birth, such as those born at high altitude or patients with cyanotic congenital heart disease. The

---

* See J. B. West: *Respiratory Physiology—The Essentials*, ed. 3, p. 40. Baltimore, Williams & Wilkins, 1985.

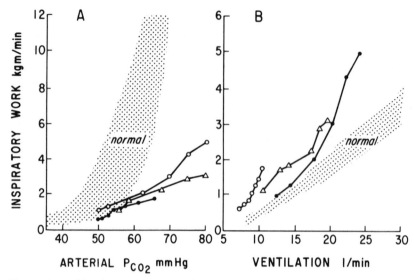

Figure 3.3. Ventilatory response to CO_2 in three patients with chronic obstructive lung disease. (*A*) They performed an abnormally small amount of inspiratory work as the inspired P_{CO_2} was raised. (*B*) They required an abnormally high work for a given level of ventilation. (From D. J. Lane and J. B. L. Howell: Relationship between sensitivity to carbon dioxide and clinical features in patients with chronic airways obstruction. *Thorax* 25:150–159, 1970 (13).)

hypoxic ventilatory response tends to be preserved during sleep. However, some patients develop sleep apnea syndromes, as discussed on page 25.

The $P_{0.1}$ response to occlusion apparently measures the total neural discharge of the respiratory center. Allowance should be made for changes in lung volume since these can affect the relationship between the stimulus to the inspiratory muscles and the pressure that they develop. The $P_{0.1}$ response to occlusion has been shown to be depressed by anesthetics and respiratory depressant drugs.

EXERCISE TESTS

Measurement

The normal lung has enormous reserves of function at rest. For example, the O_2 uptake and CO_2 output can be increased at least 10-fold when a normal subject exercises with no fall in arterial P_{O_2} or rise in P_{CO_2}. Therefore, in order to reveal minor dysfunction, the stress of exercise is often useful. Another reason for exercise testing is to assess disability. Patients vary considerably in their own assessment of the amount of activity they can do, and an objective measurement on a treadmill or stationary bicycle can be very revealing. Occasionally exercise tests are diagnostic, for example, in exercise-induced asthma or myocardial ischemia causing angina.

The variables which are often measured during exercise include work load, total ventilation, respiratory frequency, tidal volume, heart rate, ECG, blood pressure, O_2 uptake, CO_2 output, and respiratory exchange ratio. More specialized measurements such as arterial P_{O_2}, P_{CO_2}, and pH; diffusing capacity; cardiac output; and blood lactate concentration are sometimes made. Abnormal gas exchange can be characterized by the physiological dead space and shunt as at rest.

Interpretation

In most instances the interpretation of the tests on exercise is similar to that at rest except that exercise exaggerates the abnormalities. For example, a patient with interstitial lung disease who has a marginally reduced diffusing capacity at rest may show almost no increase on exercise (a very abnormal result), with a marked fall in arterial P_{O_2}, a relatively small rise in cardiac output, and perhaps striking dyspnea. Figure 3.4B shows the exercise response of a patient with hypersensitivity pneumonitis (14). Note the very rapid increase in ventilation at relatively low work levels and the fall in arterial P_{O_2} and P_{CO_2}.

Some investigators take special note of the respiratory exchange ratio (R) as the exercise level is increased, although this is technically relatively difficult to measure. When the patient reaches the limit of his steady-state aerobic exercise (anaerobic threshold), the R rises rapidly. This is caused by an increase in the CO_2 production secondary to the liberation of lactic acid from the hypoxic muscles. The hydrogen ions react with bicarbonate and lead to an increase in CO_2 excretion above that produced by aerobic metabolism. The fall in pH provides an additional stimulus to breathing.

Sometimes it is possible to identify the chief factor limiting exercise in a patient with mixed disease (15). For example, patients with both heart and lung disease present a common problem. Exercise testing may reveal that at a patient's maximum work load there is very abnormal pulmonary gas exchange with a high physiological dead space and shunt, suggesting that his lung is the weak link. Alterna-

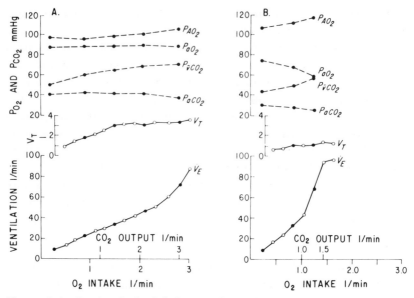

Figure 3.4. Results obtained during exercise testing. (*A*) A normal pattern. (*B*) Results in a patient with hypersensitivity pneumonitis. Note the restricted work level as evidenced by the very limited O_2 intake, the excessive ventilation for the O_2 intake, and the marked fall in arterial P_{O_2}. (From N. L. Jones: Exercise testing in pulmonary evaluation. *N. Engl. J. Med.* 293:541–544, 647–650, 1975 (14).)

tively, his cardiac output may respond poorly to exercise, thus suggesting heart disease as the chief culprit. Sometimes, however, the interpretation is not clear-cut.

DYSPNEA

This is a convenient place to briefly consider one of the most important symptoms of lung disease. *Dyspnea* refers to the sensation of difficulty with breathing and should be distinguished from simple tachypnea (rapid breathing) or hyperpnea (increased ventilation). Because dyspnea is a subjective phenomenon it is difficult to measure, and the factors responsible for it are poorly understood. Broadly speaking, dyspnea occurs when the *demand for ventilation* is out of proportion to the patient's *ability to respond* to that demand. As a result, breathing becomes difficult, uncomfortable, or labored.

An *increased demand for ventilation* is often caused by changes in the blood gases and pH. High ventilations on exercise are commonly seen in patients with inefficient pulmonary gas exchange, especially those with large physiological dead spaces, who tend to develop CO_2 retention and acidosis unless they achieve high ventilations. Another important factor is stimulation of intrapulmonary receptors. This factor presumably explains the very high exercise ventilations in many patients with interstitial lung disease possibly as a result of stimulation of the juxtacapillary (J) receptors (Figure 3.4B).

A *reduced ability to respond* to the ventilatory needs is generally caused by abnormal mechanics of the lung or chest wall. Frequently, increased airway resistance is the culprit, as in asthma, but other causes include a stiff chest wall, as in kyphoscoliosis.

The assessment of dyspnea is difficult. Usually exercise tolerance is determined from a standard questionnaire which grades breathlessness according to how far the patient can walk on the level or up stairs without pausing for breath. Occasionally ventilation is measured at a standard level of exercise and then related to the patient's maximum voluntary ventilation in an attempt to obtain an index of dyspnea. However, it should be remembered that dyspnea is something that only the patient feels and as such cannot be accurately measured.

TOPOGRAPHICAL DIFFERENCES OF LUNG FUNCTION

Measurement

The regional distribution of blood flow and ventilation in the lung can be measured with radioactive substances. The commonest method of detecting areas of absent blood flow is by injection of albumin aggregates labeled with radioactive technetium or iodine. An image of the radioactivity is then made with a gamma camera or scanner and "cold" areas containing no activity are readily apparent. The major application of this method in practice is the diagnosis of pulmonary embolism.

The distribution of blood flow can also be obtained from an intravenous injection of radioactive xenon dissolved in saline. When the gas reaches the pulmonary capillaries, it is evolved into the alveolar gas, and the radiation can be detected by a gamma camera or a series of counters. This method has the advantage that it gives blood flow per unit volume of lung.

The distribution of ventilation can be measured in a similar way, except that the gas is inhaled into the alveoli from a spirometer. Either a single inspiration or a washin over a series of breaths can be recorded. Again, ventilation per unit volume of lung is available.

Interpretation

The distribution of blood flow in the upright lung is uneven, being much greater at the base than the apex (Figure 3.5). The differences are caused by gravity and can be explained by the relationships between the pulmonary arterial, venous, and alveolar pressures.* Exercise results in a more uniform distribution because of the increase in pulmonary arterial pressure, and the same result is found in disease conditions such as pulmonary hypertension and left-to-right cardiac shunts. Increased pulmonary venous pressure, for example in mitral stenosis, initially causes a more even distribution. However, later in the disease apical flow may exceed basal flow (Figure 6.6). The mechanism of this is uncertain, though interstitial edema may play a role. Localized lung disease, for example, a cyst, or area of fibrosis, frequently decreases regional blood flow.

The distribution of ventilation is also gravity-dependent, and normally the ventilation to the base exceeds that to the apex. The explanation is the distortion which the lung suffers because of gravity and the larger transpulmonary pressure at the apex compared with the base.* Localized lung disease, for example, a bulla, usually reduces the ventilation in that area. In generalized lung disease such as asthma, chronic bronchitis and emphysema, and interstitial fibrosis, areas of reduced ventilation and blood flow can frequently be detected.

Normal subjects show a reversal of the normal pattern of ventilation if they inhale a small amount of radioactive gas from residual volume. The reason is that the airways at the base of the lung are closed under these conditions because intrapleural pressure actually rises above airway pressure. The same pattern may occur at FRC in older subjects because the lower zone airways close at an abnormally high lung volume. Similar findings may be seen in patients with emphysema, interstitial edema, and obesity. All these conditions exaggerate airway closure at the base of the lung.

Other regional differences of structure and function are also known to be present. The gravity-induced distortion of the upright lung causes the alveoli at the apex to be larger than those at the base. These larger alveoli are also associated with greater mechanical stresses which may play a role in the development of some diseases such as centrilobular emphysema (Figure 4.5A) and spontaneous pneumothorax.

* See J. B. West: *Respiratory Physiology—The Essentials*, ed. 3, p. 94. Baltimore, Williams & Wilkins, 1985.

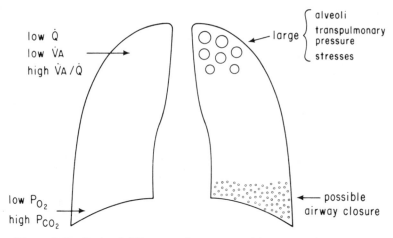

low $\dot{Q}$
low $\dot{V}A$
high $\dot{V}A/\dot{Q}$

large { alveoli
transpulmonary pressure
stresses

low P_{O_2}
high P_{CO_2}

possible airway closure

Figure 3.5.   Regional differences of structure and function in the upright lung.

VALUE OF PULMONARY FUNCTION TESTS

This book is about the function of diseased lungs and it is natural that we should start with a discussion of pulmonary function tests. However, it is important to recognize that these tests have a limited role in clinical practice. They are rarely useful in making a specific diagnosis; rather, they provide supporting information which is added to that obtained from the clinical history, physical examination, chest radiograph, and laboratory tests. Lung function tests are particularly valuable in following the progress of a patient, for example, assessing the efficacy of bronchodilator therapy in a patient with asthma. They are also useful in assessing patients for surgery, determining disability for purposes of workmen's compensation, and estimating the prevalence of disease in a community, for example, in a coal mine or an asbestos factory. It is important to appreciate that lung function tests are occasionally within normal limits in spite of obvious generalized lung disease (Figure 7.7).

As has been emphasized, spirometry gives useful information with a minimum of effort. Arterial blood gases are more difficult to measure, but the data may be lifesaving in patients with respiratory failure. The value of the other tests depends to a large extent on the particular clinical problem, and whether they are worth doing is related to the facilities of the pulmonary function laboratory.

SECTION TWO

FUNCTION OF THE DISEASED LUNG

4. Obstructive diseases

5. Restrictive diseases

6. Vascular diseases

7. Occupational and other diseases

This section is devoted to the patterns of abnormal function in the common types of lung disease.

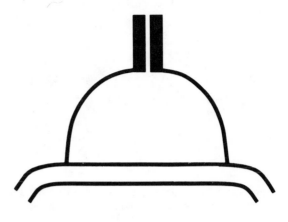

chapter **4**

Obstructive Diseases

Obstructive diseases of the lung are extremely common. In the United States they are second only to heart disease as a cause of disability benefits under Social Security. They are also becoming increasingly important as a cause of mortality. Unfortunately, as we shall see, the distinction between the various types of obstructive diseases is blurred and this gives rise to difficulties in definition and diagnosis. However, all these diseases are characterized by airway obstruction.

AIRWAY OBSTRUCTION

Increased resistance to airflow can be caused by conditions (A) inside the lumen, (B) in the wall of the airway, and (C) in the peribronchial region (Figure 4.1).

A. The lumen may be partially occluded by excessive secretions such as in chronic bronchitis. Partial obstruction may also occur acutely in pulmonary edema or following aspiration of fluids, and postoperatively with retained secretions. Inhaled foreign bodies may cause localized partial or complete obstruction.

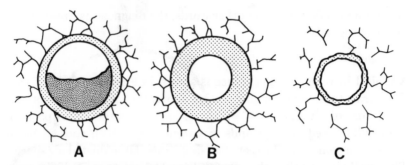

Figure 4.1. Mechanisms of airway obstruction. (*A*) The lumen is partly blocked, for example, by excessive secretions. (*B*) The airway wall is thickened, for example, by edema or muscle hypertrophy. (*C*) The abnormality is outside the airway; in the example shown, the lung parenchyma is partly destroyed and the airway has narrowed because of loss of radial traction.

B. Causes in the wall of the airway include contraction of bronchial smooth muscle as in asthma, hypertrophy of the mucous glands as in chronic bronchitis (Figure 4.6), and inflammation and edema of the wall as in bronchitis and asthma.

C. Outside the airway, destruction of lung parenchyma may cause loss of radial traction and consequent narrowing as in emphysema. A bronchus may also be locally compressed by an enlarged lymph node or neoplasm. Peribronchial edema can also cause narrowing (Figure 6.5).

CHRONIC OBSTRUCTIVE LUNG DISEASE

This is an ill-defined term which is often applied to patients who have emphysema, chronic bronchitis, or a mixture of the two. There are many patients who complain of increasing shortness of breath over several years and are found to have a chronic cough, poor exercise tolerance, evidence of airway obstruction, overinflated lungs, and impaired gas exchange. It is often difficult to know to what extent these patients have emphysema or chronic bronchitis, and the term "chronic obstructive lung disease" is a convenient nondescript label which avoids the necessity of making an unwarranted diagnosis with inadequate data.

Emphysema

This is characterized by enlargement of the air spaces distal to the terminal bronchiole, with destruction of their walls. Note that this is an anatomical definition; in other words, the diagnosis is presumptive in the living patient.

Pathology

A typical histological appearance is shown in Figure 4.2*B*. Note that in contrast to the normal lung section above, the emphysematous lung shows loss of alveolar walls with consequent destruction of parts of the capillary bed (16). Strands of parenchyma which contain blood vessels can sometimes be seen coursing across large dilated air spaces. The small airways (less than 2 mm diameter) are narrowed, tortuous, and reduced in number. In addition, they have thin, atrophied walls. There is also some loss of larger airways. The structural changes are well seen with the naked eye or hand lens in large slices of lung (Figure 4.3).

Types

Various types of emphysema are recognized. The definition given above indicates that the disease affects the parenchyma distal to the terminal bronchiole. This unit is the acinus or primary lobule, but it may not be uniformly damaged. In *centrilobular emphysema* the destruction is limited to the central part of the lobule, and the peripheral alveolar ducts and alveoli may escape unscathed (Figure 4.4). By contrast, *panlobular emphysema* shows distension and destruction of the whole lobule. Occasionally the disease is most marked in lung adjacent to interlobular septa (*paraseptal emphysema*). In other patients, large cystic areas or bullae develop (*bullous emphysema*).

Centrilobular and panlobular emphysema tend to have different topographical distributions. The former is typically most marked in the apex of the upper lobe but spreads down the lung as the disease progresses (Figure 4.5*A*). The predilection for the apex might reflect the higher mechanical stresses (Figure 3.5), which predispose to structural failure of the alveolar walls. By contrast, panlobular emphysema has no regional preference, or possibly is more common in the lower lobes. When emphysema is severe it is difficult to distinguish the two types, which may co-exist in the same lung. The centrilobular form is extremely common, and mild forms apparently cause no dysfunction.

Another form of emphysema is that associated with α_1-*antitrypsin deficiency*. Patients who are homozygous for the Z gene frequently develop severe panlobular emphysema, which usually begins in the

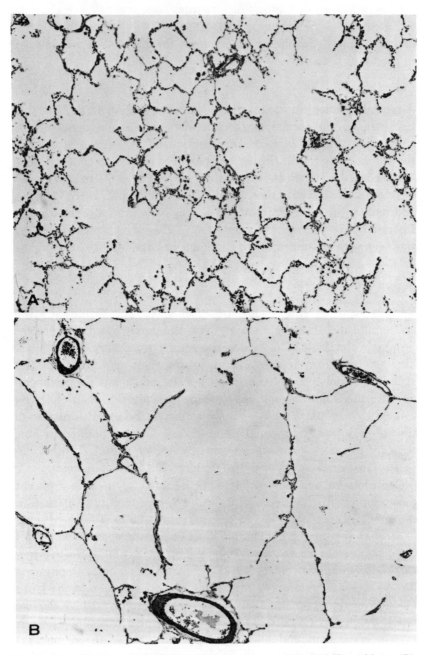

Figure 4.2. Microscopic appearance of emphysematous lung. (*A*) Normal lung. (*B*) Loss of alveolar walls and consequent enlargement of air-spaces (× 90). (From B. E. Heard: *Pathology of Chronic Bronchitis and Emphysema.* London, Churchill, 1969 (16).)

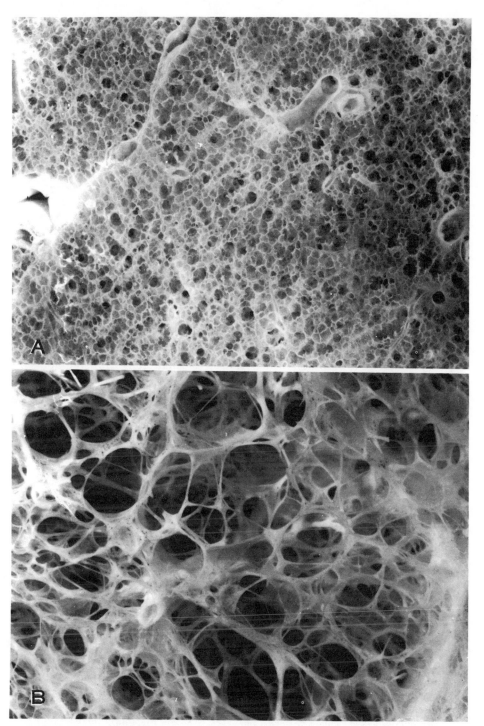

Figure 4.3. Appearance of slices of normal and emphysematous lung. (*A*) Normal. (*B*) Panlobular emphysema (barium sulfate impregnation, × 14). (From B. E. Heard: *Pathology of Chronic Bronchitis and Emphysema.* London, Churchill, 1969 (16).)

NORMAL   CENTRILOBULAR   PANLOBULAR

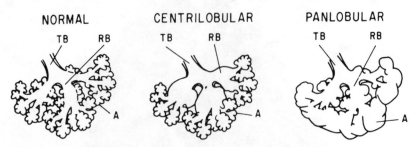

Figure 4.4. Centrilobular and panlobular emphysema. Note that in centrilobular emphysema, the destruction is confined to the terminal and respiratory bronchioles (TB and RB). In panlobular emphysema the peripheral alveoli (A) are also involved.

lower lobes (Figure 4.5B) (17). The disease may become evident by the age of 40 years and often occurs without cough or smoking history. Therapy by replacement of α_1-antitrypsin may soon be possible. Heterozygotes do not seem to be at risk, although this is not certain. Other variants of emphysema include unilateral emphysema (MacLeod's or Swyer-James' syndrome), which causes a unilaterally transradiant chest radiograph.

Etiology

The mechanisms of development of this common condition are still not well understood. Certainly cigarette smoking is an important causative factor, possibly as a result of the release of proteases from leukocytes and macrophages. However, other factors must also be important because some heavy smokers do not develop the disease. Air pollution may play a role, and hereditary factors are clearly important in the emphysema of α_1-antitrypsin deficiency.

Chronic Bronchitis

This disease is characterized by excessive mucus production in the bronchial tree, sufficient to cause excessive expectoration of sputum. Note that this is a clinical definition (unlike the definition of emphy-

---

Figure 4.5. Topographic distribution of emphysema. (A) The typical upper zone preference of centrilobular emphysema. (B) The typical lower zone preference of emphysema caused by α_1-antitrypsin deficiency. (From B. E. Heard: *Pathology of Chronic Bronchitis and Emphysema.* London, Churchill, 1969 (16); and C. Mittman (ed.): *Pulmonary Emphysema and Proteolysis.* New York, Academic Press, 1972 (17).)

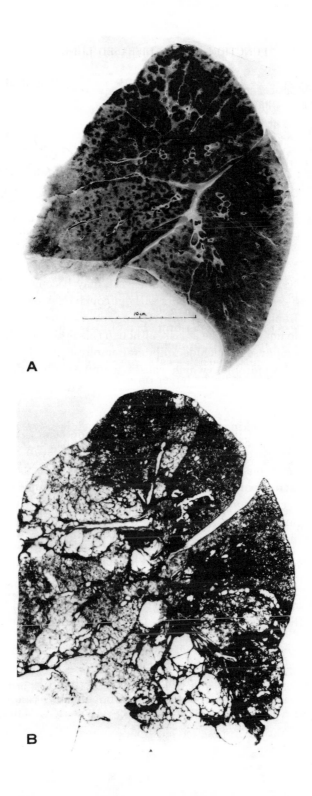

A

B

sema). In practice, criteria for "excessive" expectoration are often laid down, for example, expectoration on most days for at least 3 months in the year for at least 2 successive years.

Pathology

The hallmark is hypertrophy of mucous glands in the large bronchi (Figure 4.6) and evidence of chronic inflammatory changes in the small airways (18). The mucous gland enlargement may be expressed as the gland/wall ratio, which is normally less than 0.4 but may exceed 0.7 in severe chronic bronchitis. This is known as the Reid index (Figure 4.7). Excessive amounts of mucus are found in the airways, and semi-solid plugs of mucus may occlude some small bronchi.

In addition, the small airways are narrowed and show inflammatory changes including cellular infiltration and edema of the walls. Granulation tissue is present and peribronchial fibrosis may develop. There is apparently an increase in bronchial smooth muscle. There is some evidence that the initial pathological changes are in the small airways and that these progress to the larger bronchi.

Etiology

Again, cigarette smoking is the chief culprit. If you hear a patient give a fruity cough, you can safely bet that he is a smoker. Air pollution caused by smog or industrial smoke is another definite factor.

Clinical Features of Chronic Obstructive Lung Disease

As we have seen, chronic bronchitis is a clinical definition and the diagnosis in the living patient can therefore be made confidently. However, a definitive diagnosis of emphysema requires histological confirmation and this is usually not available during life. It follows that the amount of emphysema which is present in a given patient is uncertain and this is why chronic obstructive lung disease remains a useful term.

Within the spectrum of chronic obstructive lung disease, two extremes of clinical presentation are recognized, type A and type B. At one time it was thought that these correlated with the relative amounts of emphysema and chronic bronchitis respectively, in the lung, but more recent work shows that the situation is more complicated. Nevertheless, the terms are still useful to describe two patterns of clinical presentation. In practice most patients have features of both.

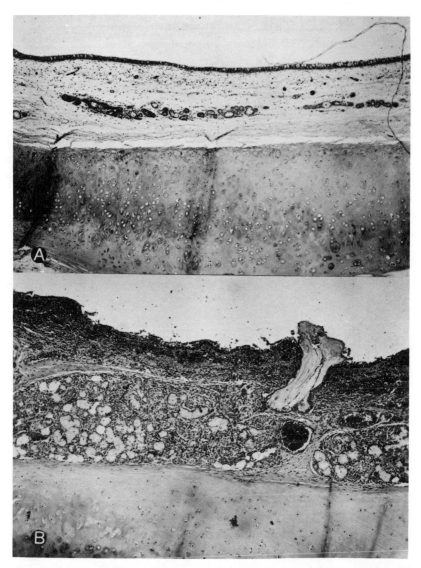

Figure 4.6. Histologic changes in chronic bronchitis. (*A*) A normal bronchial wall. (*B*) That of a patient with chronic bronchitis. Note the great hypertrophy of the mucous glands, the thickened submucosa, and the cellular infiltration (× 60). Compare with the diagram of the bronchial wall in Figure 4.7. (From W. M. Thurlbeck: *Chronic Airflow Obstruction in Lung Disease*. Philadelphia, W. B. Saunders, 1976 (18).)

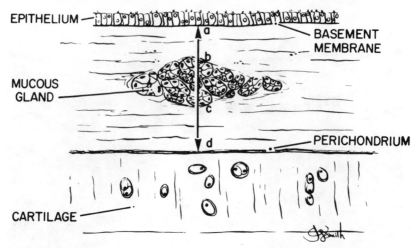

Figure 4.7. Structure of a normal bronchial wall. In chronic bronchitis the thickness of the mucous glands increases and can be expressed as the Reid index given by (b − c)/(a − d). (From W. M. Thurlbeck: *Chronic Airflow Obstruction in Lung Disease.* Philadelphia, WB Saunders, 1976 (18).)

Type A

A typical presentation would be a man in his middle 50's who has had increasing shortness of breath for the last 3 or 4 years. Cough may be absent or productive of little white sputum. Physical examination reveals an asthenic build with evidence of recent weight loss. The chest is over-expanded with quiet breath sounds and no adventitious sounds. The radiograph (Figure 4.8*B*) confirms the overinflation with low, flat diaphragms, narrow mediastinum, and increased retrosternal translucency (between the sternum and the heart on the lateral view). In addition, the radiograph shows attenuation and narrowing of the peripheral pulmonary vessels. At autopsy, extensive panlobular emphysema is a typical finding. These patients have been dubbed "pink puffers."

Figure 4.8. Radiographic appearance in emphysema. (*A*) Normal lung. (*B*) The pattern of overinflation, with low flat diaphragms, narrow mediastinum, and increased translucency which is seen in emphysema. The original film also showed attenuation and narrowing of the peripheral pulmonary vessels, but these details do not reproduce well.

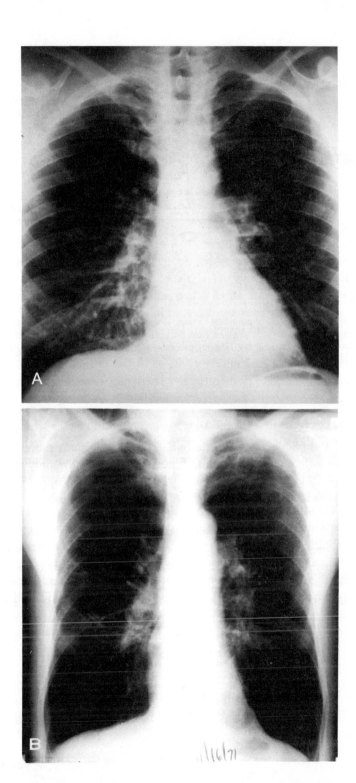

Type B

A typical presentation would be a man in his 40's with a history of chronic cough with expectoration for several years. This has gradually increased in severity, being present only in the winter months initially but more recently lasting most of the year. Acute exacerbations with frankly purulent sputum have become more common. Shortness of breath on exertion has gradually worsened, with progressively limiting exercise tolerance. The patient is almost invariably a cigarette smoker of many years' duration.

On examination, the patient has a stocky build with a plethoric complexion and some cyanosis. Auscultation reveals scattered rales and rhonchi. There may be signs of fluid retention with a raised jugular venous pressure and ankle edema. The chest radiograph shows some cardiac enlargement, congested lung fields, and increased markings attributable to old infection. Parallel lines ("tram lines") may be seen, probably caused by the thickened walls of inflamed bronchi. At autopsy, chronic inflammatory changes in the bronchi are the rule if the patient had severe bronchitis, but there may be severe emphysema as well. These patients are sometimes called "blue-bloaters."

Pathological Basis of Types A and B

As indicated above, it was initially believed that type A patients had predominantly emphysema while type B patients had mainly chronic bronchitis. Recent work (18) shows this notion is too simple. Part of the confusion is that different criteria for the two types have been used by different physicians. Naturally, if we restrict the type B classification to patients with severe chronic cough with expectoration, as in the original description (19), such patients are likely to show the pathological features of chronic bronchitis. However, the extent of the emphysema in the lung is difficult to predict during life.

Some physicians believe that the essential difference between the two types is in the control of breathing. They suggest that the more severe hypoxemia and consequent higher evidence of cor pulmonale in the type B patients can be attributed to a reduced ventilatory drive, especially during sleep.

Other Terms for Chronic Obstructive Lung Disease

Other terms such as "chronic airflow obstruction" (18) and "chronic airflow limitation" have been introduced. Part of the stimulus to use new names is to avoid some of the preconceptions associated with the old terms and to encourage fresh thinking. Also the term "obstructive" may imply a blockage within the airway to some people, but as we have seen this does not explain the reduced airflow in emphysema (Figure 4.1C). However, these new terms themselves are not well defined as yet; for example, sometimes they include asthma, and sometimes not.

Pulmonary Function

Most of the features of disordered function in chronic obstructive lung disease follow from the pathologic features discussed above and illustrated in Figures 4.2 to 4.7.

Ventilatory Capacity and Mechanics

The forced expiratory volume in 1 sec ($FEV_{1.0}$), vital capacity (VC), forced expiratory volume as a percentage of vital capacity (FEV/FVC %), forced expiratory flow ($FEF_{25-75\%}$), and maximum expiratory flow at 50% and 75% of vital capacity ($\dot{V}_{max_{50\%}}$ and $V_{max_{75\%}}$) are all reduced. All of these measurements reflect the airway obstruction, whether this is caused by excessive mucus in the lumen or thickening of the wall by inflammatory changes on the one hand (Figure 4.1A and B) or loss of radial traction on the other (Figure 4.1C). The VC is reduced because the airways close prematurely at an abnormally high lung volume, giving an increased residual volume (RV). Again, all three mechanisms of Figure 4.1 may be contributing factors.

Examination of the spirogram shows that the flow rate over most of the forced expiration is greatly reduced and the *expiratory time* is much increased. Indeed, some physicians regard this prolonged time as an excellent simple bedside index of obstruction. Often the maneuver is terminated by breathlessness when the patient is still exhaling. The low flow rate over most of the forced expiration partly reflects the reduced elastic recoil of the emphysematous lung, which generates the pressure responsible for flow under these conditions of dynamic compression (Figure 1.6). Typically the $FEV_{1.0}$ may be reduced to less than 0.8 liters in severe disease (normal value is about 4 liters in young healthy males). Note that the normal values are very dependent on age, height, weight, and sex (see Appendix).

In some patients the $FEV_{1.0}$, VC, and FEV/FVC % may increase significantly following the administration of a bronchodilator aerosol (e.g., 1% isoproterenol by nebulizer for 3 min). Such reactive airways are particularly likely to be found in a bronchitic during an exacerbation of infection. Marked response to bronchodilators over a period of weeks suggests asthma, and this disease may overlap with chronic bronchitis.

The flow-volume curve is grossly abnormal in severe disease. Figure 1.8 shows that after a brief interval of moderately high flow, flow is strikingly reduced as the airways collapse and flow limitation by dynamic compression occurs. A scooped-out appearance is often seen. Flow is greatly reduced in relation to lung volume and ceases at a high lung volume because of premature airway closure (Figure 1.5B).

The total lung capacity (TLC), functional residual capacity (FRC), and residual volume (RV) are all typically increased in emphysema. Often the RV/TLC % may exceed 40% (less than 30% in young normals). There is often a striking discrepancy between the FRC determined by the body plethysmograph on the one hand and the gas dilution techniques (helium equilibration or N_2 washout) on the other, the former being higher by 1 liter or even more. This may be caused by regions of uncommunicating lung behind grossly distorted airways. However, often the disparity reflects the slow equilibration process in very poorly ventilated areas. These static lung volumes are also often abnormal in chronic bronchitis, although the increases in volume are generally less marked. In chronic obstructive lung disease, the increased FRC and RV occur because of both the reduced lung elastic recoil and the abnormalities in the airways.

Elastic recoil of the lung is reduced in emphysema (Figure 3.1), the pressure-volume curve being displaced up and to the left. This change reflects the disorganization and perhaps loss of elastic tissue as a result of destruction of alveolar walls. The transpulmonary pressure at TLC is low. In uncomplicated chronic bronchitis in the absence of emphysema, the pressure-volume curve may be normal since the parenchyma is little affected.

Airway resistance (related to lung volume) is increased in chronic obstructive lung disease. All the factors shown in Figure 4.1 may be responsible. However, it is possible to distinguish between an increased resistance caused by intrinsic narrowing of the airway or debris in the lumen (Figure 4.1A and B) on the one hand and loss of elastic recoil and radial traction (Figure 4.1C) on the other. This can be done by relating resistance to the static elastic recoil (compare Figure 1.9).

Figure 4.9 shows airway conductance (reciprocal of resistance) plotted against static transpulmonary pressure in a series of 10 normal subjects, 10 patients with emphysema (without bronchitis), and 10 asthmatics (20). The measurements were made during a quiet, unforced expiration. Note that the relationship between conductance and transpulmonary pressure for the patients with emphysema was almost normal. In other words, we can ascribe their reduced ventilatory capacity almost entirely to the effects of the smaller elastic recoil pressure of the lung. This not only reduces the effective driving pressure during a forced expiration but also allows the airways to collapse more easily because of loss of radial traction. The small displacement of the emphysematous line to the right probably reflects the distortion and loss of airways in this disease.

By contrast, the line for the asthmatics shows that the airway conductance was greatly reduced at a given recoil pressure. Thus, the higher resistance in these patients can be ascribed to intrinsic narrowing of the airways caused chiefly by contraction of smooth muscle. After inhalation of a bronchodilator drug, isoproterenol, the asthmatic line moved toward the normal position (not shown in Figure 4.9). Comparable data are not available for a group of patients with chronic bronchitis without emphysema because it is virtually impossible to

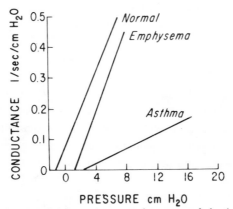

Figure 4.9. Relationships between airway conductance and elastic recoil pressure in obstructive lung disease. Note that the line for emphysema lies close to the normal line. This is evidence that any increase in airway resistance is chiefly caused by the smaller elastic recoil of the lung. By contrast, in asthma, the line is markedly abnormal due to the intrinsic narrowing of the airways. (From H. J. H. Colebatch, K. E. Finucane, and M. M. Smith: Pulmonary conductance and elastic recoil relationships in asthma and emphysema. *J. Appl. Physiol.* 34:143–153, 1973 (20).)

select such a group during life. However, Figure 4.9 clarifies the behavior of different types of airway obstruction.

Gas Exchange

Ventilation-perfusion inequality is inevitable in chronic obstructive lung disease, and this leads to hypoxemia with or without CO_2 retention. Typically, the type A patient has only moderate hypoxemia (P_{O_2} often in the high 60's or 70's) and the arterial P_{CO_2} is normal. By contrast, the type B patient often has severe hypoxemia (P_{O_2} often in the 50's or 40's) with an increased P_{CO_2}, especially in advanced disease.

The alveolar-arterial difference for P_{O_2} is always increased, especially in patients with severe bronchitis. A Riley analysis (Figure 2.9) reveals increases in both physiological dead space and physiological shunt. The dead space is particularly increased in emphysema, while high values for shunt are especially common in bronchitics.

The reasons for these differences are clarified by results obtained with the inert gas elimination technique (Figure 2.10). Figure 4.10 shows a typical distribution in a patient with advanced type A disease (21). This 76-year-old man had a history of increasing dyspnea over

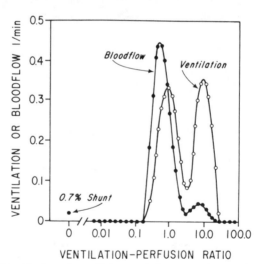

Figure 4.10. Distribution of ventilation-perfusion ratios in a patient with type A chronic obstructive lung disease. Note the large amount of ventilation to units with high ventilation-perfusion ratios (physiological dead space). (From P. D. Wagner, D. R. Dantzker, R. Dueck, J. L. Clausen, and J. B. West: Ventilation-perfusion inequality in chronic pulmonary disease. *J. Clin. Invest.* 59:203–206, 1977 (21).)

several years. The chest radiograph showed hyperinflation with atten-
uated small pulmonary vessels. The arterial P_{O_2} and P_{CO_2} were 68 and
39 mm Hg, respectively.

The distribution shows that a large amount of ventilation went to
lung units with very high ventilation-perfusion ratios ($\dot{V}_A/\dot{Q}$) (compare
Figure 2.10). This would be shown as physiological dead space in the
Riley analysis and is largely wasted from the point of view of gas
exchange. By contrast there is little blood flow going to units with an
abnormally low $\dot{V}_A/\dot{Q}$. This explains the relatively mild degree of
hypoxemia in the patient and the fact that the calculated physiological
shunt was only slightly increased.

These findings can be contrasted with those shown in Figure 4.11,
which shows the distribution in a 47-year-old man with advanced
chronic bronchitis and type B disease. He was a heavy smoker and
had had a productive cough for many years. The arterial P_{O_2} and P_{CO_2}
were 47 and 50 mm Hg respectively. Note that there was some increase
in ventilation to high $\dot{V}_A/\dot{Q}$ units (physiological dead space). However,
the distribution chiefly shows large amounts of blood flow to low
$\dot{V}_A/\dot{Q}$ units (physiological shunt), accounting for his severe hypoxemia.

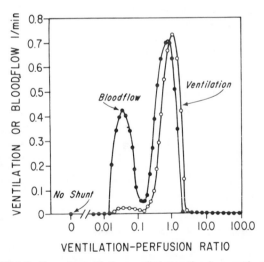

Figure 4.11. Distribution of ventilation-perfusion ratios in a patient with type B
chronic obstructive lung disease. There is a large amount of blood flow to units with
very low ventilation-perfusion ratios (physiological shunt). (From P. D. Wagner, D. R.
Dantzker, R. Dueck, J. L. Clausen, and J. B. West: Ventilation-perfusion inequality in
chronic pulmonary disease. *J. Clin. Invest.* 59:203–206, 1977 (21).)

It is remarkable that there was no blood flow to unventilated alveoli (true shunt). Indeed, true shunts of more than a few per cent are uncommon in chronic obstructive lung disease. Note that though patterns shown in Figures 4.10 and 4.11 are typical, considerable variation is seen in patients with chronic obstructive lung disease.

On exercise, the arterial P_{O_2} may fall or rise. The changes depend on the response of the ventilation and the cardiac output, and the changes in distribution of ventilation and blood flow. In some patients at least, the main factor in the fall of P_{O_2} is the limited cardiac output which, in the presence of ventilation-perfusion inequality, exaggerates any hypoxemia. Patients with CO_2 retention often show higher P_{CO_2} values on exercise because of their limited ventilatory response.

The reasons for the ventilation-perfusion inequality are clear when we consider the disorganization of the lung architecture in emphysema (Figures 4.2 and 4.3) and the abnormalities in airways in chronic bronchitis (Figure 4.6). There is ample evidence of uneven ventilation as determined by single breath tests and multibreath washouts. The latter are often reported as showing a large group of poorly ventilated alveoli and a small group of very well-ventilated alveoli. However, in practice, there is probably a spectrum of ventilations from very low to very high values. Topographical measurements with radioactive xenon show regional inequality of both ventilation and blood flow. The blood flow inequality is largely caused by destruction of portions of the capillary bed. In addition, there is some hypertrophy of smooth muscle in the walls of the small pulmonary arteries in advanced disease, which may contribute to the nonuniformity of flow.

An unresolved question is to what extent the inequality of ventilation in chronic obstructive lung disease is of the parallel or series type (Figure 1.11). The essential lesion of centrilobular emphysema is dilatation of the respiratory bronchioles in the middle of the acinus (Figure 4.4), and this is certainly one morphological abnormality which could cause series inequality. However, we do not yet know how important this mechanism is in practice.

The deleterious effects of airway obstruction on gas exchange are reduced by the collateral ventilation which occurs in these patients. Communicating channels normally exist between adjacent alveoli and between neighboring small airways (22), and there have been many experimental demonstrations of these. The fact that there is so little blood flow to unventilated units in these patients (Figures 4.10 and 4.11) emphasizes the effectiveness of collateral ventilation, since some airways must presumably be completely closed, especially in severe bronchitis (Figure 1.11).

Another factor which reduces the amount of ventilation-perfusion inequality is hypoxic vasoconstriction.* This local response to a low alveolar P_{O_2} reduces the blood flow to poorly ventilated and unventilated regions, minimizing the arterial hypoxemia. When patients with chronic obstructive lung disease are given bronchodilators, for example, isoproterenol, they sometimes develop a slight fall in arterial P_{O_2}. This is probably caused by the vasodilator action of these β-adrenergic drugs, increasing the blood flow to poorly ventilated areas. This finding is more marked in asthma (see below).

The arterial P_{CO_2} is often normal in patients with mild to moderate chronic obstructive lung disease in spite of their ventilation-perfusion inequality. This is because any tendency for the arterial P_{CO_2} to rise stimulates the chemoreceptors, thus increasing ventilation to the alveoli (Figure 2.11). As disease becomes more severe, the arterial P_{CO_2} may rise. This is particularly likely to occur in type B patients. The increased work of breathing is an important factor, but there is also evidence that the sensitivity of the respiratory center to CO_2 is reduced in some of these patients (see below).

If the arterial P_{CO_2} rises, the pH tends to fall, resulting in respiratory acidosis. In some patients the P_{CO_2} rises so slowly that the kidney is able to compensate adequately by retaining bicarbonate and the pH remains almost constant (compensated respiratory acidosis). In other instances, the P_{CO_2} rises more suddenly, perhaps as a consequence of an acute chest infection. Under these conditions acute respiratory acidosis may occur (see Chapter 8).

Additional information about gas exchange can be obtained in these patients by measuring the diffusing capacity (transfer factor) for carbon monoxide (Figure 2.13). The diffusing capacity as measured by the single breath method is particularly likely to be reduced in patients with severe emphysema. By contrast, patients with chronic bronchitis but little parenchymal destruction often have normal values.

These results must be interpreted cautiously. Emphysematous lungs

* See J. B. West: *Respiratory Physiology—The Essentials*, ed. 3, p. 43. Baltimore, Williams & Wilkins, 1985.

have lost much of their alveolar surface and thus the area available for diffusion, and the capillary blood volume are reduced. However, it is difficult to know how far the measurement of diffusing capacity reflects this because of the degree of unevenness of ventilation, blood flow, and diffusing properties. Such lungs empty very unevenly and the small post-dead space sample which is analyzed will probably not be representative of the lung as a whole. Thus, the diffusing capacity is best regarded as an empirical index of impaired gas transfer with few or no implications about the morphology of the blood-gas barrier.

Pulmonary Circulation

The pulmonary artery pressure frequently rises in patients with chronic obstructive pulmonary disease as their disease progresses. Several factors are responsible. In emphysema large portions of the capillary bed are destroyed, thus increasing vascular resistance. Hypoxic vasoconstriction also raises the pulmonary arterial pressure, and often an exacerbation of chest infection causes an additional transient increase as the hypoxia worsens. In advanced disease, histological changes in the walls of the small arteries occur. Finally, these patients often develop polycythemia as a response to the hypoxemia, and this increases blood viscosity. This occurs most commonly in patients with severe bronchitis, who tend to have the lowest arterial P_{O_2}.

Fluid retention with dependent edema and engorged neck veins may occur, especially in the type B patients. The right heart often enlarges, with characteristic radiologic and electrocardiographic appearances. The term cor pulmonale is given to this condition, but whether it should be regarded as right heart failure is disputed. The output of the heart is normally increased because it is operating high on the Starling curve, and the output can rise further on exercise.

Control of Ventilation

As indicated above, some patients with chronic obstructive lung disease, particularly those with severe chronic bronchitis, develop CO_2 retention because they do not sufficiently increase the ventilation to their alveoli. The reasons why some patients behave in this way and some do not are not completely understood. One factor is the increased work of breathing as a result of the high airway resistance. As a consequence, the O_2 cost of breathing may be enormous (Figure 4.12) (23). It is known that normal subjects have an abnormally small

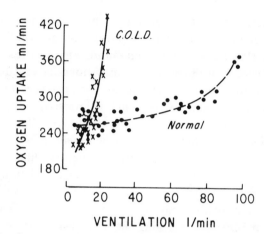

Figure 4.12. Oxygen uptake during voluntary hyperventilation in patients with chronic obstructive lung disease (C.O.L.D.). Note the very high values compared with those of the normal subjects. (From R. M. Cherniak, L. Cherniak, and A. Naimark: *Respiration in Health and Disease*, ed. 2. Philadelphia, W. B. Saunders, 1972 (23).)

ventilatory response to inhaled CO_2 if a resistance is attached to the mouthpiece.* Thus, a patient with a severely limited O_2 consumption may be willing to forgo a normal arterial P_{CO_2} to obtain the advantage of a reduced work of breathing and a correspondingly reduced O_2 cost. However, the correlation between airway resistance and arterial P_{CO_2} is sufficiently poor that some other factor must be involved.

Measurements of the ventilatory response to inhaled CO_2 and of the pressure generated during a brief inspiratory obstruction show that there are marked differences between normal subjects. These are partly due to personality, genetic, and racial factors. Some patients can be shown to have a reduced respiratory center output in response to inhaled CO_2, many have a mechanical obstruction to ventilation, and some patients have both (Figure 3.3). Thus, it is possible that the ventilatory response which a patient makes in the face of severe ventilation-perfusion inequality and an increased work of breathing is predetermined to some extent by these factors.

Changes in Early Disease

So far we have mainly been concerned with pulmonary function in patients with well-established disease. However, relatively little can

---

* See J. B. West: *Respiratory Physiology—The Essentials*, ed. 3, p. 122. Baltimore, Williams & Wilkins, 1985.

be done to reverse the disease process in this group, and the management is limited chiefly to prevention and control of infection, relief of bronchoconstriction, and general rehabilitative measures. Therefore, there is a great deal of current interest in identifying patients with early disease in the hope that the changes can be arrested or reversed. At the very least, these patients could be strongly advised to stop smoking.

It was emphasized earlier that since relatively little of the airway resistance resides in small airways (less than 2 mm diameter), pathological changes there may go unnoticed by the usual function tests. Some physicians believe that the earliest changes in chronic obstructive lung disease probably occur in these small airways. Tests of small airway function which are currently being assessed include the FEV, $FEF_{25-75\%}$, $\dot{V}_{max_{50\%}}$, and $\dot{V}_{max_{75\%}}$, flow-volume curve during helium breathing, closing volume, and dynamic compliance. The practical value of these tests for the early detection of disease is still uncertain.

ASTHMA

This disease is characterized by increased responsiveness of the airways to various stimuli and manifested by widespread narrowing of the airways that changes in severity, either spontaneously or as a result of treatment.

Pathology

The airways have hypertrophied smooth muscle which contracts during an attack, causing bronchoconstriction (Figure 4.1B). In addition, there is hypertrophy of mucous glands, edema of the bronchial wall, and extensive infiltration by eosinophils (Figure 4.13). The mucus is abnormal; it is thick, tenacious, and slow-moving. Many of the airways are occluded by mucous plugs, some of which may be coughed up in the sputum (Curschmann's spirals). The sputum is typically scant and white. In uncomplicated asthma there is no destruction of alveolar walls and there are no copious purulent bronchial secretions. Occasionally the abundance of eosinophils in the sputum gives it a purulent appearance, which may be wrongly ascribed to infection.

Mechanism of Bronchoconstriction

Rapid progress is being made in this area (24, 25). The following account will no doubt be modified and should be regarded as a working

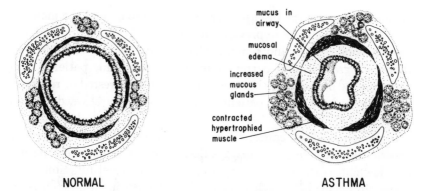

Figure 4.13. Bronchial wall in asthma (diagrammatic). Note the hypertrophied, contracted smooth muscle, edema, mucous gland hypertrophy, and secretion in the lumen.

hypothesis. The tone of smooth muscle cells is apparently controlled by the intracellular level of cyclic AMP, decreased levels causing contraction. In response to an extrinsic antigen, immunoglobulin IgE is produced by plasma cells and lymphoid tissue and binds to mast cells in the bronchial walls (Figures 4.14 and 4.15). The antigen-antibody reaction which then occurs on the surface of the mast cell results in the release of mediator substances, some of which are stored in the granules of the mast cells. The release of the mediators also may be modulated by the intracellular levels of cyclic AMP and GMP. β-Adrenergic agents increase cyclic AMP levels, resulting in decreased mediator release, while cholinergic agents may decrease cyclic AMP levels or increase cyclic GMP levels, thus increasing release. The mediators include histamine, slow-reacting substance of anaphylaxis (SRS-A), now known to be one or more leukotrienes, eosinophilic chemotactic factor (ECF-A), prostaglandins, bradykinin, and others. Many of these mediators react at specific receptor sites on the membranes of the smooth muscle cells and thereby cause a reduction in the intracellular level of cyclic AMP. This results in contraction of the smooth muscle. The mediators also increase capillary permeability, resulting in edema. Other mechanisms such as changes in levels of intracellular calcium may also contribute to the action of these mediators.

The autonomic nervous system also plays a role. Stimulation of receptors in the bronchial wall, possibly as a result of the release of

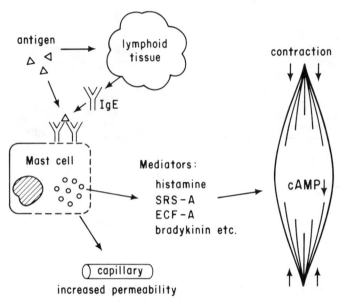

Figure 4.14. Mechanism of bronchoconstriction in asthma. (See text for details.)

mediators, causes reflex bronchoconstriction via the vagus nerve. This can be blocked by atropine. The heightened response of the parasympathetic nervous system may explain why the airways of asthmatics are sensitive to nonspecific irritants. In addition, this mechanism may be important in asthmatics who do not have increased IgE levels in their blood.

An additional factor in asthmatics may be a relative insensitivity of the β-adrenergic receptors of the bronchial smooth muscle. When stimulated, these increase the level of cyclic AMP and thus cause bronchodilation. The β-receptors may be insensitive because of low levels of synthesis of receptors, because of antibodies directed against receptors, or because of altered coupling between receptors and adenyl cyclase.

Clinical Features

Asthma begins commonly in children but may occur at any age. There is frequently a family history. The patient may have a previous history to suggest atopy, including hay fever, eczema, or urticaria, and may relate the asthmatic attacks to a specific pollen for example, ragweed.

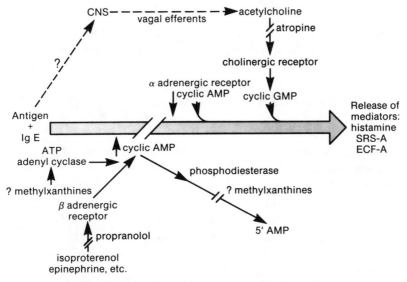

Figure 4.15. Regulation of mediator release in asthma.

Such a patient is said to have extrinsic asthma. If there is no general history of allergy and no external allergen can be identified, the term intrinsic asthma is sometimes used.

There is usually evidence of general hyperreactivity of the airways, with the result that nonspecific irritants such as smog bring on an attack. Psychological factors are often important, and attacks may follow exercise, especially in a cold environment. Aspirin ingestion is a cause in some individuals. Between attacks the patient may have no symptoms.

During the attack the patient may be extremely dyspneic, orthopneic, agitated, and confused. The accessory muscles of respiration are active. The lungs are hyperinflated and musical wheezes are heard in all areas. The pulse is rapid and pulsus paradoxicus may be present (marked fall in systolic and pulse pressure during inspiration). The sputum is scant and viscid. The chest radiograph reveals hyperinflation but is otherwise normal.

Status asthmaticus refers to an attack which continues for hours or even days without remission. There are often signs of exhaustion, dehydration, and marked tachycardia. The chest may become ominously silent, and vigorous treatment is urgently required.

Bronchodilators

Drugs which reverse or prevent bronchoconstriction play a major role in the management of patients with asthma. They are also useful in those patients with chronic bronchitis who have some reversible airway obstruction.

Bronchodilator drugs include the following.

β-Adrenergic Agonists

These include isoproterenol, isoetharine, metaproterenol, terbutaline, and salbutamol. These drugs stimulate β-adrenergic receptors in bronchial smooth muscle, increasing the activity of adenyl cyclase and thus raising the level of cyclic AMP (Figure 4.15). β-Adrenergic receptors are of two types: β_1 receptors exist in the heart and elsewhere, and their stimulation increases heart rate and the force of contraction of cardiac muscle. Stimulation of β_2 receptors relaxes smooth muscle in the bronchi, blood vessels, and uterus.

Isoproterenol is an effective, widely used bronchodilator which is given as an aerosol. However, it is both a β_1 and β_2 agonist and so may cause unwanted tachycardia and palpitations. Terbutaline, metaproterenol, and salbutamol are believed to mainly stimulate the β_2 receptors and thus cause fewer side effects.

Methylxanthines

These include aminophylline and theophylline. These drugs increase cyclic AMP by inhibiting the enzyme phosphodiesterase, an enzyme which breaks down cyclic AMP. In addition, other mechanisms such as increased release of adrenal catecholamines and blockade of adenosine receptors probably contribute to the efficacy of methylxanthines as bronchodilators. Measurement of blood levels is an aid to determining the correct dose. Aminophylline can be given intravenously during a severe attack of asthma.

Corticosteroids

These include prednisolone and beclomethasone. The action of these drugs in asthma is not fully understood, but they reduce inflammatory changes and edema and may also increase the level of cyclic AMP in the bronchial smooth muscle, thus causing relaxation. They are best reserved for patients who fail to respond to other drugs.

Parasympatholytic Agents

Atropine is an example. There is evidence that the parasympathetic nervous system plays a part in the asthma reaction, but these drugs are currently little used in the United States because of their side effects. Newer agents that may avoid these side effects are under development.

Cromolyn Sodium

This useful drug is not a bronchodilator, but it is effective in the prophylaxis of allergic asthma. It is given by inhalation. Its mode of action is uncertain, but it appears to stabilize the mast cell, preventing the release of mediators (Figure 4.14). The drug is not useful during an attack, but if it is given before challenge with an antigen, the attack is averted.

Beclomethasone Dipropionate

This is a corticosteroid preparation which is given by inhalation. It is not a bronchodilator, but it is very effective in preventing attacks of allergic asthma. The drug appears to act locally in the respiratory tract, with the absorption of relatively little into the circulation; thus, systemic side effects, a major problem with oral corticosteroids, do not occur. However, oral *Candida* infections may develop.

Pulmonary Function

As was the case with chronic bronchitis and emphysema, the changes in lung function generally follow clearly from the pathology of asthma.

Ventilatory Capacity and Mechanics

During an attack, all indices of expiratory flow rate are markedly reduced, including the $FEV_{1.0}$, FEV/FVC %, $FEF_{25-75\%}$, $\dot{V}_{max_{50\%}}$, and $\dot{V}_{max_{75\%}}$. The VC is also usually reduced because airways close prematurely toward the end of a full expiration. Between attacks some impairment of ventilatory capacity can usually be demonstrated.

The response of these indices to bronchodilator drugs is of great importance in asthma (Figure 4.16). This may be tested by administering 1% isoprenaline by aerosol for 2 min. Typically, all indices increase substantially when a bronchodilator is administered to a patient during an attack, and the change is a valuable measure of the

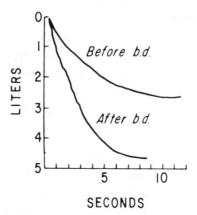

SECONDS

Figure 4.16. Examples of forced expirations before and after bronchodilator (b.d.) therapy in a patient with bronchial asthma. Note the striking increase in flow rate and vital capacity. (From D. V. Bates, P. T. Macklem, and R. V. Christie: *Respiratory Function in Disease*, ed. 2. Philadelphia, W. B. Saunders, 1971 (9).)

responsiveness of the airways. The extent of the increase varies according to the severity of the disease. In status asthmaticus, very little change may be seen because the bronchi have become unresponsive. Again, patients in remission may show only minor improvement, though there is generally some.

There is some evidence that the relative change in $FEV_{1.0}$ and FVC following bronchodilator therapy indicates whether the bronchospasm has been completely relieved. During an asthma attack, both the $FEV_{1.0}$ and FVC tend to increase by the same fraction, with the result that the FEV/FVC % remains low and almost constant. However, when the tone of the airway muscle is nearly normal, the $FEV_{1.0}$ responds more than the FVC, and the FEV/FVC % approaches the nromal value of about 75%.

The flow-volume curve in asthma has the typical obstructive pattern, although it may not exhibit the scooped out appearance seen in emphysema. After a bronchodilator, flows are higher at all lung volumes and the whole curve may shift as the TLC and RV are reduced.

Static lung volumes are increased, and remarkably high values for FRC and TLC during asthma attacks have been reported. The increased RV is caused by premature airway closure during a full expiration as a result of the increased smooth muscle tone, edema and inflammation of the airway walls, and abnormal secretions. The cause of the increased FRC and TLC is not fully understood. However, there is some loss of elastic recoil and the pressure-volume curve is shifted upward and to the left (Figure 3.1). This tends to return toward normal following a bronchodilator. There is some evidence that changes in the surface tension of the alveolar lining layer may be responsible for the altered elastic properties. The rise in lung volume tends to decrease resistance of the airways by increasing their radial traction. The FRC measured by helium dilution is usually considerably below that found with the body plethysmograph, reflecting the presence of occluded airways or the very delayed equilibration of poorly ventilated areas.

Airway resistance as measured in the body plethysmograph is raised, and it falls following a bronchodilator. It is likely that the bronchospasm affects airways of all sizes, and the relationship between airway conductance and elastic recoil pressure is markedly abnormal (Figure 4.9). Narrowing of the large and medium-sized bronchi can be seen directly at bronchoscopy.

Gas Exchange

Arterial hypoxemia is common in asthma and is caused by ventilation-perfusion ($\dot{V}A/\dot{Q}$) inequality. There is ample evidence of uneven ventilation, both by single breath and multibreath washout methods. In addition, measurements with radioactive xenon show regions of reduced ventilation, especially when these are sought by recording the washin or washout rate of the gas. Marked topographical inequality of blood flow is also seen and, typically, different areas show transient reductions at different times. Both physiological dead space and physiological shunt are generally abnormally high.

An example of a distribution of ventilation-perfusion ratios in a 47-year-old asthmatic is shown in Figure 4.17. This patient had only mild symptoms at the time of the measurement. The distribution is markedly different from the normal distribution shown in Figure 2.10. Note especially the bimodal distribution, with a considerable amount of the total blood flow (about 25%) going to units with a very low $\dot{V}A/\dot{Q}$ (about 0.1). This accounts for the patient's mild hypoxemia, the arterial P_{O_2} being 81 mm Hg. There is no pure shunt (blood flow to unventilated alveoli), a surprising finding in view of the mucous plugging of airways which is a feature of the disease.

When this patient was given the bronchodilator isoproterenol by

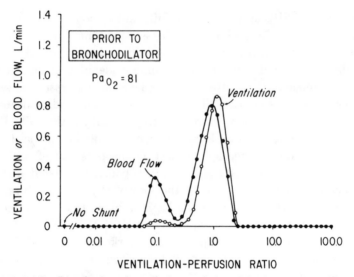

Figure 4.17. Distribution of ventilation-perfusion ratios in a patient with asthma. Note the bimodal appearance, with about 25% of the total blood flow going to units with ventilation-perfusion ratios in the region of 0.1.

aerosol, there was an increase in $FEF_{25-75\%}$ from 3.4 to 4.2 liters/sec. Thus, there was some relief of his bronchospasm. The changes in the distribution of ventilation-perfusion ratios are shown in Figure 4.18. Note that the blood flow to the low $\dot{V}A/\dot{Q}$ alveoli increased from about 25 to 50% of the total flow resulting in a fall in arterial P_{O_2} from 81 to 70 mm Hg. The mean $\dot{V}A/\dot{Q}$ of the low mode increased slightly from 0.10 to 0.14, indicating that the ventilation to these units increased slightly more than their blood flow. Again no shunt was seen.

Many bronchodilators decrease the arterial P_{O_2} in asthmatics, including isoproterenol, aminophylline, and terbutaline. An exception is orciprenaline. The mechanism of the increased hypoxemia is apparently relief of vasoconstriction in poorly ventilated areas. This vasoconstriction probably results from the release of mediators, like the bronchoconstriction. The fall in P_{O_2} is accompanied by increases in physiological shunt and dead space. However, in practice the favorable effects of the drugs on airway resistance far exceed the disadvantages of the mild additional hypoxemia.

The absence of shunt—that is, blood flow to unventilated lung units—in Figures 4.17 and 4.18 is striking, especially since asthmatics

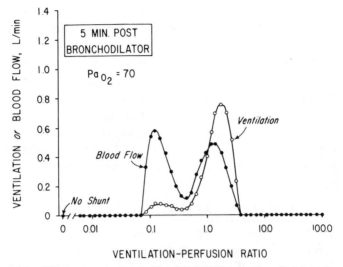

Figure 4.18. The same patient as in Figure 4.17, following the administration of the bronchodilator isoproterenol by aerosol. Note the increase in blood flow to the units with low ventilation-perfusion ratios and the corresponding fall in arterial P_{O_2}.

who come to autopsy have mucous plugs in some of their airways. Presumably, the explanation is collateral ventilation which reaches lung situated behind completely closed bronchioles. This is shown diagrammatically in figure 1.11. The same mechanism probably exists in the lungs of patients with chronic bronchitis (see Figure 4.11 for example).

The arterial P_{CO_2} in patients with asthma is typically normal or low, at least until very late in the disease. The P_{CO_2} is prevented from rising by increased ventilation to the alveoli in the face of the ventilation-perfusion inequality (compare Figure 2.11). In many patients the P_{CO_2} may be in the middle or low 30's, possibly as a result of stimulation of the peripheral chemoreceptors by the mild hypoxemia or stimulation of intrapulmonary receptors.

In status asthmaticus the arterial P_{CO_2} may begin to rise and the pH to fall. This is an ominous development which denotes impending respiratory failure and signals the need for urgent and intensive treatment. Mechanical ventilation may be necessary (Chapter 10). Deaths from asthma have apparently increased in recent years, and respiratory failure is one cause. Another may be ventricular fibrillation caused by the abuse of inhalers containing drugs with β_1-adrenergic effects. These may cause an abnormal rhythm in a hypoxic myocardium.

The diffusing capacity for carbon monoxide is typically normal or high in uncomplicated asthma. If it is reduced, associated emphysema should be suspected. The reason for the increased diffusing capacity is probably the large lung volume. Hyperinflation increases the diffusing capacity in normal subjects, presumably by increasing the area of the blood-gas interface. Following bronchodilators, the diffusing capacity falls in asthmatics, partly because of worsening of the ventilation-perfusion relationships.

LOCALIZED AIRWAY OBSTRUCTION

So far this chapter has been devoted to generalized airway obstruction, both irreversible as in emphysema and chronic bronchitis and reversible as in asthma. Localized obstruction is less common and generally causes less functional impairment. Obstruction may be within the lumen of the airway, in the wall, or as a result of compression from outside the wall (Figure 4.1).

Tracheal Obstruction

This can be caused by an inhaled foreign body, scarring following trauma or surgery, or compressing masses such as an enlarged thyroid. There are inspiratory and expiratory stridor, reduced maximum flow rates in both inspiration and expiration, and no response to bronchodilators. Hypoventilation may result in hypercapnia and hypoxemia (Figures 2.3 and 2.4).

Bronchial Obstruction

This is often caused by a foreign body, for example an inhaled peanut. The right lung is more frequently affected than the left, because the left main bronchus makes a sharper angle with the trachea than the right. Other common causes are bronchial tumors, either malignant or benign, and compression of a bronchus by enlarged surrounding lymph nodes. This last particularly affects the right middle lobe bronchus because of its anatomical relationships.

If obstruction is complete, absorption atelectasis occurs because the sum of the partial pressures in mixed venous blood is less than in alveolar gas.* The collapsed lobe is often visible on the radiograph, where compensatory overinflation of adjacent lung and displacement of a fissure may be seen. Perfusion of the unventilated lung is reduced because of hypoxic vasoconstriction and also the increased vascular resistance caused by the mechanical effects of the reduced volume on the extra-alveolar vessels and the capillaries. However, the residual blood flow contributes to hypoxemia. The most sensitive test is the alveolar-arterial P_{O_2} difference during 100% O_2 breathing (Figure 2.8). Infection may follow localized obstruction and lead to lung abscess. If the obstruction is in a segmental or smaller bronchus, atelectasis may not occur because of collateral ventilation (Figure 1.11).

* See J. B. West: *Respiratory Physiology—The Essentials*, ed. 3, p. 135. Baltimore, Williams & Wilkins, 1985.

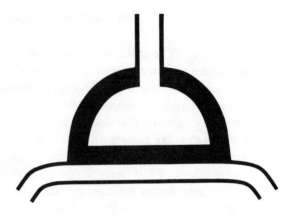

chapter **5**

Restrictive Diseases

Restrictive diseases are those in which the expansion of the lung is restricted either because of alterations in the lung parenchyma or because of disease of the pleura, the chest wall, or the neuromuscular apparatus. They are characterized by a reduced vital capacity and a small resting lung volume (usually), but the airway resistance (related to lung volume) is not increased. These diseases are therefore very different from the obstructive diseases in their pure form, although mixed restrictive and obstructive conditions can occur.

DISEASES OF THE LUNG PARENCHYMA

This term refers to the alveolar tissue of the lung and a brief review of the structure of this is pertinent.

Structure of the Alveolar Wall

Figure 5.1 shows an electron micrograph of a pulmonary capillary in an alveolar wall (26). The various structures through which oxygen passes on its way from the alveolar gas to the hemoglobin of the red blood cell are pulmonary surfactant (not shown in this preparation),
92

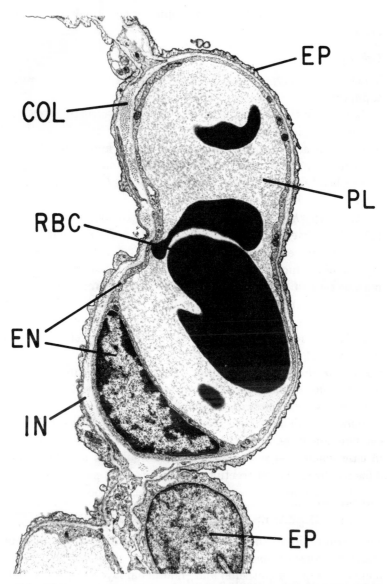

Figure 5.1. Electron micrograph of portion of an alveolar wall. *EP*, epithelium; *COL*, collagen; *PL*, plasma; *RBC*, red blood cell; *EN*, endothelial cell; *IN*, interstitium (× 6300). (From E. R. Weibel: Morphological basis of alveolar-capillary gas exchange. *Physiol. Rev.* 53:419–495, 1973 (26).)

alveolar epithelium, interstitium, capillary endothelium, plasma, and erythrocyte.

Cell Types

The various cell types have different functions and different responses to injury.

Type 1 Epithelial Cell. This is the chief structural cell of the alveolar wall; its long protoplasmic extensions pave almost the whole alveolar surface (Figure 5.1). The cell has no known functions apart from mechanical support. It rarely divides and is not very active metabolically. When type 1 cells are injured, they are replaced by type 2 cells, which later transform into type 1.

Type 2 Epithelial Cell. This is a nearly globular cell (Figure 5.2) (27) which gives little structural support to the alveolar wall but is metabolically very active. The electron micrograph shows the lamellated bodies which contain phospholipid. This is formed in the endoplasmic reticulum, passed through the Golgi apparatus, and eventually extruded into the alveolar space to form surfactant.* Following injury to the alveolar wall, these cells rapidly divide to line the surface and then later transform into type 1 cells. A type 3 cell has also been described but it is rare and its function is unknown.

Alveolar Macrophage. This scavenger cell roams around the alveolar wall phagocytosing foreign particles and bacteria. The cell contains lysozymes which digest engulfed foreign matter.

Fibroblast. This cell synthesizes collagen and elastin, which are components of the interstitium of the alveolar wall. Following various disease insults, large amounts of these materials may be laid down. This results in interstitial fibrosis.

Interstitium

This fills the space between the alveolar epithelium and the capillary endothelium. Figure 5.1 shows that it is very thin on one side of the capillary, where it essentially consists of a fusion of the basement membranes of the epithelial and endothelial layers. On the other side of the capillary, the interstitium is usually wider and includes fibrils of collagen. It is possible that the thick side is chiefly concerned with

---

*See J. B. West: *Respiratory Physiology—The Essentials*, ed. 3, p. 91. Baltimore, Williams & Wilkins, 1985.

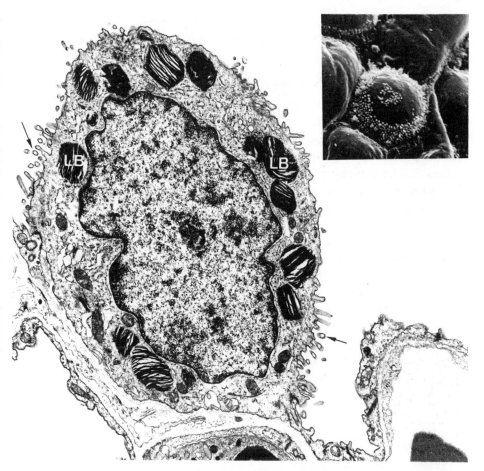

Figure 5.2. Electron micrograph of type 2 epithelial cell (× 10,000). Note the osmiophilic lamellated bodies (*LB*), large nucleus, and microvilli (*arrows*), which are mainly concentrated around the edge of the cell, and cytoplasm rich in organelles. The *inset* at *top right* is a scanning electron micrograph showing the surface view of a type 2 cell with its characteristic distribution of microvilli (× 3400). (From E. R. Weibel and J. Gil: Structure-function relationships at the alveolar level. In J. B. West (ed.): *Bioengineering Aspects of the Lung*, p. 15. New York, Marcel Dekker, 1977 (27).)

fluid exchange across the endothelium, whereas the thin side is responsible for most of the gas exchange (Figure 6.1).

Interstitial tissue is found elsewhere in the lung, notably in the perivascular and peribronchial spaces around the larger blood vessels and airways and in the interlobular septa. The interstitium of the alveolar wall is continuous with that in the perivascular spaces (Figure 6.1) and is the route by which fluid drains from the capillaries to the lymphatics.

Diffuse Interstitial Pulmonary Fibrosis

The nomenclature of this condition is confusing. Synonyms include idiopathic pulmonary fibrosis, interstitial pneumonia, intrinsic (or cryptogenic) fibrosing alveolitis, and the Hamman-Rich syndrome. Some physicians reserve the term "fibrosis" for the late stages of the disease. The changes in pulmonary function will be described in some detail because they are typical of many of the other conditions alluded to later in this chapter.

Pathology

The principal feature is thickening of the interstitium of the alveolar wall. Initially there is infiltration with lymphocytes and plasma cells. Later, fibroblasts appear and lay down thick collagen bundles (Figure 5.3) (28). These changes may be irregularly dispersed within the lung. Eventually the alveolar architecture is destroyed and the scarring results in multiple air-filled cystic spaces formed by dilated terminal and respiratory bronchioles—so-called "honeycomb lung." In some patients a cellular exudate consisting of macrophages and other mononuclear cells is seen within the alveoli. This is called "desquamation."

Etiology

Unknown, though in some cases an immunological reaction is suspected.

Clinical Features

The disease is not common and tends to affect adults in late middle age. The patient often presents with dyspnea with rapid shallow breathing. The dyspnea typically becomes very marked on exercise (compare Figure 3.4). An irritating, unproductive cough is often present.

On examination, cyanosis may be seen at rest and typically worsens on exercise. Fine crepitations are usually heard throughout both lungs, especially toward the end of inspiration. Finger clubbing is common. The chest radiograph shows a "ground glass" haziness, especially at the bases, and a generalized micronodular mottling is often present.

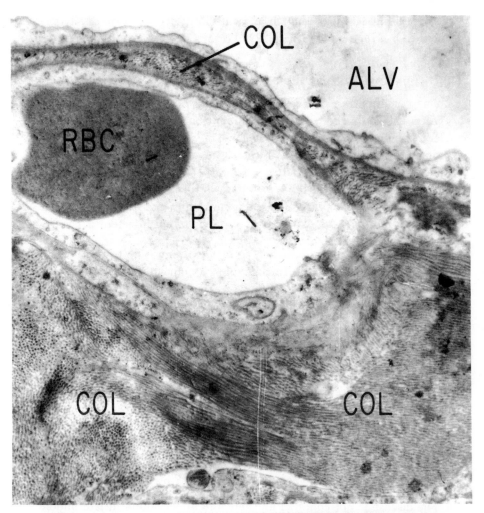

Figure 5.3.   Electron micrograph from a patient with diffuse interstitial fibrosis. Note the thick bundles of collagen. *COL*, collagen; *ALV*, alveolar space; *RBC*, red blood cell; *PL*, plasma. Compare Figure 5.1. (From D. R. Gracey, M. B. Divertie, and A. L. Brown, Jr.: Alveolar-capillary membrane in idiopathic interstitial pulmonary fibrosis. Electron microscopic study of 14 cases. *Am. Rev. Respir. Dis.* 98:16–21, 1968 (28).)

Patchy shadows near the diaphragm may be due to basal collapse. Late in the disease a honeycomb appearance is often seen; this is caused by multiple air cysts surrounded by thickened tissue.

Cor pulmonale or pneumonia may complicate the picture and the patient may develop respiratory failure terminally. The diseases often progress insidiously, although an acute form occurs as originally described by Hamman and Rich (29).

Pulmonary Function

Ventilatory Capacity and Mechanics.   Spirometry typically reveals a restrictive pattern (Figure 1.2). The VC is markedly reduced but the gas is exhaled rapidly so that although the $FEV_{1.0}$ is low, the FEV/FVC% may exceed the normal value. The almost square shape of the forced expiratory spirogram is in striking contrast to the obstructive pattern (compare Figure 4.16). The $FEF_{25-75\%}$ is normal or high. The flow-volume curve does not show the scooped out shape of obstructive disease and the flow rate is often higher than normal when related to absolute lung volume. This is shown in Figure 1.5, where it can be seen that the downslope of the curve for restrictive disease lies above the normal curve.

All lung volumes are reduced, including the TLC, FRC, and RV, but the relative proportions are more or less preserved. The pressure-volume curve of the lung is flattened and displaced downward (Figure 3.1), so that at any given volume the transpulmonary pressure is abnormally high. The maximum elastic recoil pressure which can be generated at TLC is typically higher than normal. Airway resistance is normal or low when related to lung volume.

All these results are consistent with the pathological appearance of fibrosis of the alveolar walls (Figures 2.7 and 5.3). The fibrous tissue reduces the distensibility of the lung just as a scar on the skin reduces its extensibility. As a result the lung volumes are small, and abnormally large pressures are required to distend the lung. The airways may not be specifically involved, but they tend to narrow as lung volume is reduced. However, airway resistance at a given lung volume is normal or even decreased because the retractive forces exerted on the airway walls by the surrounding parenchyma are abnormally high (Figure 5.4). The pathological correlate of this is the honeycomb appearance caused by the dilated terminal and respiratory bronchioles surrounded by thickened scar tissue.

Gas Exchange.   The arterial P_{O_2} and P_{CO_2} are typically reduced, and the pH is normal. The hypoxemia is usually mild at rest until the disease is advanced. However, on exercise the P_{O_2} often falls dramatically and cyanosis may be evident. In well-established disease both the physiological dead space and physiological shunt are increased.

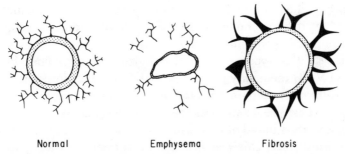

Normal   Emphysema   Fibrosis

Figure 5.4. Airway caliber in emphysema and interstitial fibrosis. In emphysema the airways tend to collapse because of the loss of radial traction. By contrast, in fibrosis, radial traction may be excessive, with the result that airway caliber is large when related to lung volume.

The relative contributions of diffusion impairment and ventilation-perfusion ($\dot{V}_A/\dot{Q}$) inequality to the hypoxemia of these patients has long been debated. It is natural to argue that the histological appearances shown in Figures 2.7 and 5.3 slow the diffusion of oxygen from the alveolar gas to the capillary blood, since the thickness of the barrier may be increased many fold (compare Figure 5.1). In addition, the increasing hypoxemia on exercise is consistent with the mechanism of impaired diffusion, since exercise reduces the time spent by the red cell in the pulmonary capillary (Figure 2.6). The term "alveolar-capillary block syndrome" was coined and has been widely applied to a variety of diseases characterized by interstitial fibrosis.

More recently, physiologists have questioned the role of impaired diffusion as the chief cause of hypoxemia in these conditions. The objections have been on two counts. First, it has been pointed out that the normal lung has enormous reserves of diffusion in that the P_{O_2} of the blood nearly reaches that in alveolar gas very early in its transit through the capillary (Figure 2.6). Second (and more important), it is clear that these patients have substantial inequality of ventilation and blood flow within the lung. Indeed, how could they not, with the disorganization of architecture shown in Figures 2.7 and 5.3? The inequalities have been demonstrated by single breath and multibreath N_2 washouts and measurements of topographical function with radioactive xenon.

In order to apportion blame for the hypoxemia between the two possible mechanisms, it is necessary to measure the degree of $\dot{V}_A/\dot{Q}$

inequality and determine how much of the hypoxemia is attributable to this. This has been done by using the multiple inert gas method in a series of patients with interstitial lung disease (30). Figure 5.5 shows that at rest, the hypoxemia could be adequately explained by the degree of $\dot{V}A/\dot{Q}$ inequality present in these patients. However, Figure 5.6 shows that on exercise, the observed alveolar P_{O_2} was consistently below the value predicted from the measured amount of $\dot{V}A/\dot{Q}$ inequality, and thus an additional cause of hypoxemia must have been present. Most likely this was diffusion impairment in these patients. However, hypoxemia caused by diffusion impairment was only evident on exercise, and even then it accounted for only about one-third of the total alveolar-arterial difference for P_{O_2}.

The low arterial P_{CO_2} in these patients (typically in the middle or low 30's) occurs in spite of the evident $\dot{V}A/\dot{Q}$ inequality and is caused by increased ventilation to the alveoli (compare Figure 2.11). The cause of the increased ventilation is uncertain. There is some evidence that the control of ventilation is abnormal because of stimulation of

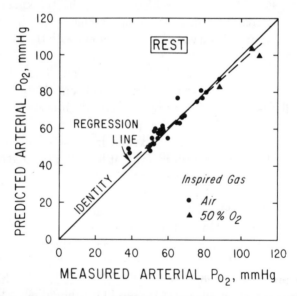

Figure 5.5. Study of the mechanism of hypoxemia in a series of patients with interstitial lung disease. This figure shows that the arterial P_{O_2} predicted from the pattern of $\dot{V}A/\dot{Q}$ inequality agreed well with the measured arterial P_{O_2}. Thus, at rest, all of the hypoxemia could be explained by the uneven ventilation and blood flow.

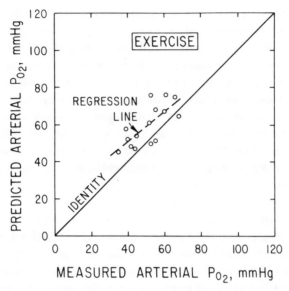

Figure 5.6.   Results obtained on exercise in the same patients as shown in Figure 5.5. Note that under these conditions the measured arterial P_{O_2} was systematically below that predicted from the pattern of $\dot{V}A/\dot{Q}$ inequality. This indicates an additional mechanism for hypoxemia, presumably diffusion impairment.

receptors within the lung (see below). Stimulation of the peripheral chemoreceptors by the arterial hypoxemia may also be a factor. The arterial pH is usually normal at rest but may increase considerably on exercise as a result of the hyperventilation and consequent respiratory alkalosis (compare Figure 3.4), though metabolic acidosis caused by lactic acid accumulation may also occur. In terminal respiratory failure, the pH may fall.

The diffusing capacity for carbon monoxide is often strikingly reduced in these patients to the neighborhood of 5 ml/min/mm Hg (normal value near 30 depending on age and stature). Indeed, this may be a useful diagnostic pointer: if the diffusing capacity is not low, the diagnosis should be regarded with suspicion. The reduction is caused in part by the thickening of the blood-gas barrier (Figure 2.7). In addition there is a fall in the blood volume of the pulmonary capillaries, since many of the vessels are obliterated by the fibrotic process. A further factor in the lower measured diffusing capacity is probably the $\dot{V}A/\dot{Q}$ inequality, which causes uneven emptying of the lung. Certainly the diffusing capacity should not be taken to reflect only the properties of the blood-gas barrier (see page 41).

Exercise.   Patients with mild diffuse interstitial fibrosis may show much more evidence of impaired pulmonary function on exercise than at rest. The changes shown in Figure 3.4*B* are typical, though this patient had extrinsic rather than intrinsic fibrosing alveolitis (see below). Note that the maximal O_2 intake and CO_2 output were severely limited compared with the normal values of Figure 3.4*A*. The increase in ventilation on exercise was markedly exaggerated. This was chiefly due to the very high rate of breathing, which rose to over 60 breaths/ min during maximal exercise.

As a result of the high ventilation, which was out of proportion to the increase in O_2 uptake and CO_2 output, the alveolar and arterial P_{CO_2} fell and the alveolar P_{O_2} rose. However, the arterial P_{O_2} fell as noted earlier, thus increasing the alveolar-arterial difference for P_{O_2}. This can be partly explained by the impaired diffusion characteristics of the lung (Figure 5.6). However, most of the hypoxemia on exercise was caused by $\dot{V}A/\dot{Q}$ inequality.

One factor which tends to reduce the arterial P_{O_2} on exercise is the abnormally small rise in cardiac output. These patients typically have some increase in pulmonary vascular resistance. This is particularly evident on exercise during which the pulmonary artery pressure may rise substantially. The high resistance can be attributed to obliteration of much of the pulmonary capillary bed by the interstitial fibrosis (Figure 2.7). Another factor is hypertrophy of vascular smooth muscle and consequent narrowing of the small arteries. It is important to appreciate that an abnormally low cardiac output in the presence of $\dot{V}A/\dot{Q}$ inequality can cause hypoxemia. One way of looking at this is to argue that a low cardiac output results in a low P_{O_2} in the mixed venous blood (page 177). As a consequence, a lung unit with a given $\dot{V}A/\dot{Q}$ will oxygenate the blood less than when the mixed venous P_{O_2} is normal.

The importance of this factor can be seen if we consider some results obtained in our laboratory in a patient with interstitial lung disease. During exercise which raised the O_2 uptake from about 300 to 700 ml/ min, the arterial P_{O_2} fell from 50 to 35 mm Hg. The rise in cardiac output was only from 4.6 to 5.7 liters/min; the normal value for this level of exercise is approximately 10 liters/min. As a result the P_{O_2} in the mixed venous blood fell to 17 mm Hg (normal value about 35 mm Hg). Calculations show that if the cardiac output had increased to 10 liters/min (and the pattern of $\dot{V}A/\dot{Q}$ inequality remained unchanged), the arterial P_{O_2} would have been some 10 mm Hg higher.

Another useful measurement during exercise in these patients is the diffusing capacity for carbon monoxide. Typically this remains low in interstitial fibrosis, whereas in normal subjects it may double or triple. These measurements must be made by the steady-state rather than the single breath method because of the difficulties of breath-holding during exercise.

Control of Ventilation. We have already seen that these patients typically have shallow rapid breathing, especially on exercise. The reason for this is not known, but it is possible that the pattern is due to reflexes originating in pulmonary irritant receptors or J (juxtacapillary) receptors. The former lie in the bronchi just under the epithelial lining and may be stimulated by the increased traction on the airways caused by the increased elastic recoil of the lung (Figure 5.4). The J receptors are in the alveolar walls and could be stimulated by the fibrotic changes in the interstitium. No direct evidence of increased activity of either receptor is yet available in man, but work in experimental animals suggests that they could cause rapid shallow breathing.

The rapid shallow pattern of breathing reduces the respiratory work in patients with a reduced lung compliance. On the other hand, it also increases ventilation of the anatomical dead space at the expense of the alveoli, so a compromise must be reached. As far as is known, no central nervous system mechanism monitors respiratory work.

Other Types of Parenchymal Restrictive Disease

The changes in pulmonary function in diffuse interstitial pulmonary fibrosis were dealt with at some length because this disease serves as a prototype for other forms of parenchymal restrictive disease. These will now be considered briefly, and differences in their pattern of pulmonary function will be discussed.

Sarcoidosis

This disease is characterized by the presence of granulomatous tissue having a characteristic histological appearance and often occurring in several organs.

Pathology.   The characteristic lesion is the epithelioid cell tubercle, composed of large histiocytes with giant cells and lymphocytes. Caseation is not present, although central hyaline degeneration may occur. In advanced pulmonary disease, fibrotic changes in the alveolar walls are seen.

Etiology.   Unknown. It is possible that the disease represents an atypical response to the tubercle bacillus or other unidentified agent.

Clinical Features.   Two patterns can be identified.

1. An acute form of the disease is seen in young people, in whom it is characterized by bilateral hilar lymph node enlargement and erythema nodosum. These may be accompanied by acute arthritis, uveitis, and parotid gland enlargement. There are no disturbances of pulmonary function in this form.

2. A chronic form of the disease is seen in the older age group. Pulmonary infiltration and fibrosis occur in the late stages. The chest radiograph shows a contracted lung with fine linear shadows and some nodulation, especially in the midzones (Figure 5.7). Cystic changes may develop, and occasionally rupture of a cyst may cause a pneumothorax. Other manifestations of the disease occur primarily in the eye, skin, bone, and kidney. A skin test (Kveim) is a valuable diagnostic aid.

Pulmonary Function.   There may be no impairment of function in the acute form of the disease until this progresses to the indolent form with pulmonary infiltration and evidence of disease in other organs. Typical changes of the restrictive type are then often seen, though the radiographic appearance sometimes suggests more interference with function than actually exists.

Ultimately, marked pulmonary fibrosis may develop, with a severe restrictive pattern of function. All lung volumes are small, but the FEV/FVC% is preserved. Lung compliance is strikingly reduced, the pressure-volume curve being flattened and shifted downward and to the right (Figure 3.1). The resting arterial P_{O_2} is low and often falls considerably on exercise. The arterial P_{CO_2} is normal or low, though terminally it may rise as respiratory failure supervenes. The diffusing capacity for carbon monoxide (transfer factor) is markedly reduced. Cor pulmonale may develop in advanced disease.

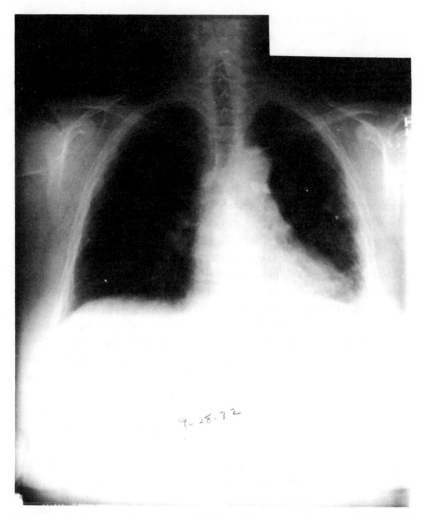

Figure 5.7. Chest radiograph of a patient with interstitial pulmonary fibrosis. Note the small contracted lung and rib cage and the raised diaphragms (compare the normal appearance in Figure 4.8*A*).

Hypersensitivity Pneumonitis

This is also known as allergic alveolitis or extrinsic fibrosing alveolitis. It is a hypersensitivity reaction affecting the lung parenchyma that occurs in response to inhaled organic dusts. The best-known example is farmer's lung. The exposure is usually occupational and heavy. The disease is an example of type 3 hypersensitivity (Arthus), and precipitins can be demonstrated in the serum.

The term "extrinsic" implies that the etiological agent is external and can be identified, in contrast to intrinsic fibrosing alveolitis (diffuse interstitial fibrosis discussed above), where the cause is unknown. Farmer's lung is due to the spores of thermophilic *Actinomyces* in moldy hay. Bird breeder's lung is caused by avian antigens from feathers and excreta. Mushroom worker's lung, maltworker's lung, and bagassosis (in sugar cane workers) are also recognized.

Pathology.   The alveolar walls are thickened and infiltrated with lymphocytes, plasma cells, and occasional eosinophils together with collections of histiocytes which in some areas form small granulomas. The small bronchioles are usually affected and there may be exudate in the lumen. Fibrotic changes occur in advanced cases.

Clinical Features.   The disease occurs in either acute or chronic forms. In the former, symptoms of dyspnea, fever, shivering, and cough appear 4–6 hr after exposure and continue for 24–48 hr. The patient is frequently dyspneic at rest, with fine crepitations throughout both lung fields. The disease may also occur in a chronic form without prior acute attacks. These patients present with progressive dyspnea, usually over a period of years. In the acute form, the chest radiograph may be normal, but frequently a miliary nodular infiltrate is present. In the chronic form, fibrosis of the upper lobes is commonly seen.

Pulmonary Function.   In well-developed disease the typical restrictive pattern is seen, as described on pages 98–103. This includes reduced lung volumes, low compliance, hypoxemia which worsens on exercise, normal or low arterial P_{CO_2}, and a reduced diffusing capacity. In the early stages variable degrees of airway obstruction may be present.

Interstitial Disease Caused by Drugs, Poisons, and Radiation

Various drugs may cause an acute pulmonary reaction, which can proceed to interstitial fibrosis. These include busulfan (used in the treatment of chronic myeloid leukemia), the antibiotic nitrofurantoin, and the cytostatic drug bleomycin. Other antineoplastic drugs can also cause fibrosis. Oxygen in high concentrations causes acute toxic changes with subsequent interstitial fibrosis (Figures 5.3 and 9.5).

Ingestion of the weedkiller, paraquat, results in the rapid development of lethal interstitial fibrosis. Therapeutic radiation which includes lung in the field causes acute pneumonitis followed by fibrosis.

Collagen Diseases

Interstitial fibrosis with a typical restrictive pattern may be found in patients with systemic sclerosis (generalized scleroderma). Dyspnea is often severe and out of proportion to the changes in radiological appearance or lung function. Other collagen diseases which may produce fibrosis include systemic lupus erythematosus and rheumatoid arthritis.

Lymphangitis Carcinomatosa

This refers to the spread of carcinoma tissue through pulmonary lymphatics and may complicate carcinomas, chiefly of the stomach or breast. Dyspnea is prominent and the typical restrictive pattern of lung function may be seen.

DISEASES OF THE PLEURA

Pneumothorax

Air can enter the pleural space either from the lung or, rarely, through the chest wall. The pressure in the intrapleural space is normally subatmospheric as a result of the elastic recoil forces of the lung and chest wall. When air enters the space, the lung collapses and the rib cage springs out.* These changes are evident on a chest radiograph (Figure 5.8), which shows partial or complete collapse of the lung, overexpansion of the rib cage and depression of the diaphragm on the affected side, and sometimes displacement of the mediastinum away from the pneumothorax. These changes are most evident if the pneumothorax is large, particularly if a tension pneumothorax is present (see below).

Spontaneous Pneumothorax

This is the commonest form and is caused by the rupture of a small bleb on the surface of the lung near the apex. It typically occurs in

---

* See J. B. West: *Respiratory Physiology—The Essentials*, ed. 3, p. 97. Baltimore, Williams & Wilkins, 1985.

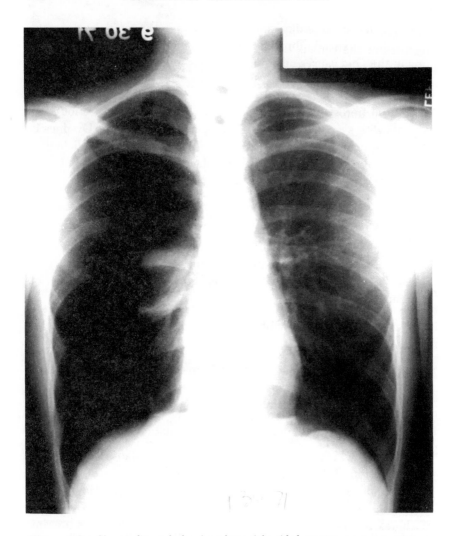

Figure 5.8. Chest radiograph showing a large right-sided spontaneous pneumothorax. Note the small, collapsed right lung, depression of the right hemidiaphragm, and overexpansion of the rib cage on the right.

tall young males and may be related to the high mechanical stresses that occur in the upper zone of the upright lung (Figure 3.5). The presenting symptom is often sudden pain on one side accompanied by dyspnea. On auscultation, breath sounds are reduced on the affected side and the diagnosis is readily confirmed by a radiograph.

The pneumothorax gradually absorbs because the sum of the partial pressures in the venous blood is considerably less than atmospheric pressure. Recurrent attacks may need surgical treatment to promote adhesions between the two pleural surfaces.

Tension Pneumothorax

In a small proportion of spontaneous pneumothoraces the communication between the lung and the pleural space functions as a check valve. As a consequence, air enters the space during inspiration but cannot escape during expiration. The result is a large pneumothorax in which the pressure may considerably exceed atmospheric pressure and thus interfere with venous return to the thorax.

This constitutes a medical emergency and is recognized by increasing respiratory distress, tachycardia, and signs of mediastinal shift such as tracheal deviation and movement of the apex beat. The radiograph is usually diagnostic. Treatment consists of relieving the pressure by inserting a tube through the chest wall. This is connected to an underwater seal which allows air to escape from the chest but not enter it.

Pneumothorax Complicating Lung Disease

This occurs in a variety of conditions including rupture of a bulla in chronic obstructive lung disease, or a cyst in advanced fibrotic disease. It also sometimes occurs during assisted ventilation with high airway pressures (see Chapter 10).

Pulmonary Function

As would be expected, a pneumothorax reduces the FEV and VC. In practice, pulmonary function tests are rarely helpful in the management of these patients because the radiograph is so informative.

Pleural Effusion

This refers to fluid rather than air in the pleural cavity. It is not a disease in its own right, but it frequently accompanies serious disease and an explanation should always be sought.

The patient often complains of dyspnea if the effusion is large, and there may be pleuritic pain from the underlying disease. The chest signs are often informative and include reduced movement of the chest on the affected side, absence of breath sounds, and dullness to percussion. The radiograph is diagnostic.

Pleural effusions can be divided into exudates and transudates according to whether their protein content is high or low. Exudates typically occur with malignancies and infections, while transudates complicate severe heart failure and other edematous states. It is often necessary to aspirate an effusion, but treatment should be directed at the underlying cause. Pulmonary function is impaired as in pneumothorax, but the measurements are not required in practice.

Variants of pleural effusion include empyema (pyothorax), hemothorax, and chylothorax, which refer to the presence of pus, blood, and lymph, respectively, in the pleural space.

Pleural Thickening

Occasionally a long-standing pleural effusion results in a rigid, contracted fibrotic pleura which splints the lung and prevents its expansion. This can result in a marked restrictive type of functional impairment, particularly if the disease is bilateral. Surgical stripping may be necessary.

DISEASES OF THE CHEST WALL

Scoliosis

Bony deformity of the chest can be a cause of restrictive disease. Scoliosis refers to lateral curvature of the spine and kyphosis to posterior curvature. Scoliosis is more serious, especially if the angulation is high in the vertebral column. It is frequently associated with a backward protuberance of the ribs, giving the appearance of an added kyphosis. In most cases the cause is unknown, though occasionally the condition is due to bony tuberculosis or neuromuscular disease.

The initial complaint is dyspnea on exertion; breathing tends to be rapid and shallow. Later, hypoxemia develops, and eventually carbon dioxide retention and cor pulmonale may supervene. Bronchitis is common if the patient smokes.

Pulmonary function tests show a reduction in all lung volumes which may be very marked. Airway resistance is nearly normal if related to lung volume. However, there is inequality of ventilation, partly because of airway closure in dependent regions. Part of the lung are compressed and there are often areas of atelectasis.

The hypoxemia is due to ventilation-perfusion inequality. In advanced disease, a reduced ventilatory response to CO_2 can often be demonstrated. This reflects the increased work of breathing caused by deformity of the chest wall. Not only is the chest wall stiff, but also the respiratory muscles operate inefficiently. The pulmonary vascular bed is restricted, causing a rise in pulmonary artery pressure, which is exaggerated by the alveolar hypoxia. Venous congestion and peripheral edema may develop. The patient may succumb to an intercurrent pulmonary infection or respiratory failure.

Ankylosing Spondylitis

In this disease of unknown etiology there is a gradual but relentless onset of immobility of the vertebral joints and fixation of the ribs. As a result, the movement of the chest wall is grossly reduced. There is a reduction of VC and TLC, but the FEV/FVC% and the airway resistance are normal. The compliance of the chest wall may fall and there is often some uneven ventilation, probably secondary to the reduced lung volume. The lung itself remains normal and diaphragmatic movement is preserved. Respiratory failure does not occur.

NEUROMUSCULAR DISORDERS

Diseases affecting the muscles of respiration or their nerve supply include poliomyelitis, Guillain-Barré syndrome, amyotrophic lateral sclerosis, myasthenia gravis, and muscular dystrophies (Figure 2.5). All these can lead to dyspnea and respiratory failure. The inability of the patient to take in a deep breath is reflected in a reduced VC, TLC, inspiratory capacity, and FEV.

It should be remembered that the most important muscle of respiration is the diaphragm, and patients with progressive disease often do not complain of dyspnea until the diaphragm is involved. By then their ventilatory reserve may be severely compromised. The progress of the disease can be monitored by measuring the VC and the blood gases. Assisted ventilation (Chapter 10) may become necessary.

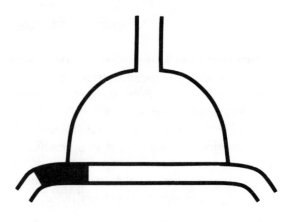

chapter 6

Vascular Diseases

PULMONARY EDEMA

This is an abnormal accumulation of fluid in the extravascular spaces and tissues of the lung. It is an important complication of a variety of heart and lung diseases and may be life-threatening.

Pathophysiology

Figure 5.1 reminds us that the pulmonary capillary is lined by endothelial cells and surrounded by an interstitial space. There is some evidence that this interstitium is very narrow on one side of the capillary, where it is formed essentially by the fusion of the two basement membranes, while on the other side it is wider and contains collagen fibers. This latter region may be particularly important for fluid exchange. Between the interstitial and alveolar spaces is the alveolar epithelium, composed predominantly of type 1 cells, and the superficial layer of surfactant (not shown in Figure 5.1).

The capillary endothelium is apparently highly permeable to water and to many solutes including small molecules and ions. Proteins have a restricted movement across the cells. By contrast, the alveolar

112

epithelium is much less permeable (except to water), and even small ions are largely prevented from crossing.

Hydrostatic forces tend to move fluid out of the capillary into the interstitial space, while osmotic forces tend to keep it in. The movement of fluid is governed by Starling's equation:

$$\dot{Q} = K[(P_c - P_i) - \sigma(\pi_c - \pi_i)]$$

where $\dot{Q}$ is the net flow out of the capillary, K is the filtration coefficient, Pc and Pi are the hydrostatic pressures in the capillary and interstitial space, respectively, π_c and π_i are the corresponding colloid osmotic pressures, and σ is the reflection coefficient. The last indicates the effectiveness of the membrane in preventing (reflecting) the passage of the protein compared with that of water across the endothelium, and the coefficient is reduced in diseases which damage the cells and increase the permeability.

Although this equation is valuable conceptually, its practical use is limited. Of the four pressures, only one, the colloid osmotic pressure within the capillary, is known with any certainty. Its value is about 28 mm Hg. The capillary hydrostatic pressure is probably about halfway between arterial and venous pressures but varies markedly from top to bottom of the upright lung. The colloid osmotic pressure of the interstitial fluid is not known but is approximately 20 mm Hg in lung lymph. However, there is some question whether this lymph has the same protein concentration as the interstitial fluid around the capillaries. The interstitial hydrostatic pressure is unknown and is thought by some physiologists to be substantially below atmospheric pressure. It is probable that the net pressure is outward, causing a lymph flow of perhaps 20 ml/hr (31).

The fluid which leaves the capillaries moves within the interstitial space of the alveolar wall and tracks to the perivascular and peribronchial interstitium (Figure 6.1). This tissue normally forms a thin sheath around the pulmonary arteries, veins, and bronchi and contains the lymphatics. The alveoli themselves are apparently devoid of lymphatics, but once the fluid reaches the perivascular and peribronchial interstitium, some of it is carried in the lymphatics while some moves through the loose interstitial tissue. The lymphatics actively pump the lymph toward the bronchial and hilar nodes.

If excessive amounts of fluid leak from the capillaries, two factors

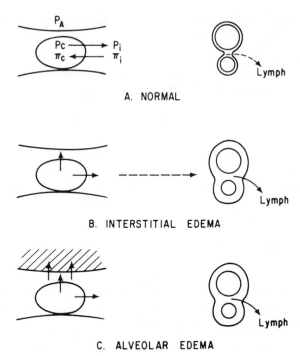

A. NORMAL

B. INTERSTITIAL EDEMA

C. ALVEOLAR EDEMA

Figure 6.1. Stages of pulmonary edema. (*A*) There is normally a small lymph flow from the lung. (*B*) Interstitial edema. Here there is an increased flow with engorgement of the perivascular and peribronchial spaces and some widening of the alveolar wall interstitium. (*C*) Some fluid crosses the blood-gas barrier, producing alveolar edema.

tend to limit this flow. The first is a fall in the colloid osmotic pressure of the interstitial fluid as the protein is diluted as a result of the faster filtration of water compared with protein. However, this factor does not operate if the permeability of the capillary is greatly increased. The second is a rise in hydrostatic pressure in the interstitial space, which reduces the net filtration pressure. Both factors act in a direction to reduce fluid movement out of the capillaries.

Two stages in the formation of pulmonary edema are recognized (Figure 6.1). The first is *interstitial edema*, which is characterized by engorgement of the perivascular and peribronchial interstitial tissue (cuffing), as shown in Figure 6.2. Widened lymphatics can be seen, and lymph flow increases. In addition, some widening of the interstitium of the alveolar wall occurs. Pulmonary function is little affected

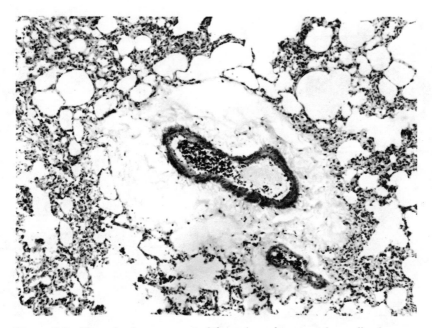

Figure 6.2. Example of engorgement of the perivascular space of a small pulmonary blood vessel by interstitial edema. Some alveolar edema is also present.

at this stage and the condition is difficult to recognize, although some radiologic changes may be seen (see below).

The second stage is *alveolar edema* (Figure 6.3) (32). Here fluid moves across into the alveoli, which are filled one by one. As a result of surface tension forces, the edematous alveoli shrink in size. Ventilation is prevented, and to the extent that the alveoli remain perfused, hypoxemia is inevitable. The edema fluid may move into the small and large airways and be coughed up as voluminous frothy sputum. In congestive heart failure, this is pink in color because of the presence of red blood cells. What prompts the transition from interstitial to alveolar edema is not fully understood, but it may be that the lymphatics become overloaded and the pressure in the interstitial space increases so much that fluids spills over into the alveoli. Probably the alveolar epithelium is damaged and its permeability is increased. This would explain the presence of protein and red cells in the alveolar fluid.

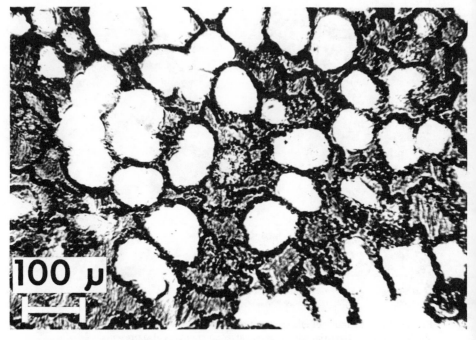

Figure 6.3. Section of dog lung showing alveolar edema. Note that some alveoli are filled completely while others are spared. The edematous alveoli tend to be smaller. (From N. C. Staub: The pathophysiology of pulmonary edema. *Hum. Pathol.* 1:419–432, 1970 (32).)

Etiology

This is best discussed under six headings (33), as shown in Table 6.1.

Increased Capillary Hydrostatic Pressure

This is the commonest cause and frequently complicates heart disease such as acute myocardial infarction, hypertensive left ventricular failure, and mitral valve disease. In all of these conditions, left atrial pressure rises, causing an increase in pulmonary venous and capillary pressures. This can be recognized at cardiac catheterization by measuring the "wedge" pressure (the pressure in a catheter that has been wedged in a small pulmonary artery), which is approximately equal to pulmonary venous pressure.

Whether pulmonary edema occurs in these conditions depends on the rate of rise of the pressure. For example, in patients with mitral

Table 6.1. Causes of Pulmonary Edema.

Mechanism	Precipitating Event
Increased capillary hydrostatic pressure	Myocardial infarction, mitral stenosis, fluid overload, pulmonary veno-occlusive disease
Increased capillary permeability	Inhaled or circulating toxins, radiation, oxygen toxicity, adult respiratory distress syndrome
Lymphatic insufficiency	Silicosis, lymphangitis carcinomatosa
?Decreased interstitial pressure	Rapid removal of pleural effusion or pneumothorax, hyperinflation
Decreased colloid osmotic pressure	Overtransfusion, hypoproteinemia
Unknown etiology	High altitude, heroin, neurogenic

stenosis in whom the venous pressure is gradually raised over a period of years, remarkably high values may occur without clinical evidence of edema. This is partly because the caliber or number of the lymphatics increases to accommodate the higher lymph flow. However, these patients often have marked interstitial edema. By contrast, a patient with an acute myocardial infarction may develop alveolar edema with a smaller but more sudden rise in venous pressure.

Noncardiogenic causes also occur. Edema may be precipitated by excessive intravenous infusions of saline, plasma or blood, leading to a rise in capillary pressure. Diseases of the pulmonary veins such as pulmonary veno-occlusive disease may also result in edema.

The cause of the edema in all these conditions is partly the increase in hydrostatic pressure per se and also probably an increased permeability of the capillaries. This is apparently due to stretching or rupturing of the endothelial lining as a result of the rise in capillary pressure.

Increased Capillary Permeability

This occurs in a variety of conditions. Toxins which are inhaled, such as chlorine, sulfur dioxide, or nitrogen oxides, or which circulate, such as alloxan or endotoxin, cause pulmonary edema in this way. Therapeutic radiation to the lung may cause edema and ultimately interstitial fibrosis. Oxygen poisoning produces a similar picture. Another cause is the adult respiratory distress syndrome (see Chapter 8).

Lymphatic Insufficiency

This occurs in diseases such as silicosis, where the normal lymphatic drainage is slowed because of obliteration or distortion of lymphatics. In lymphangitis carcinomatosa, the lymphatics are obstructed by tumor cells. Lymphatic insufficiency is also seen following lung transplantation.

Decreased Interstitial Pressure

This would be expected to promote edema from the Starling equation, though whether this occurs in practice is uncertain. However, patients who have a large unilateral pleural effusion or pneumothorax and whose lung is rapidly expanded sometimes develop pulmonary edema on that side. This may be partly related to the large mechanical forces acting on the interstitial space as the lung is expanded.* There is also evidence of some change in permeability in these patients.

Decreased Colloid Osmotic Pressure

This is rarely responsible for pulmonary edema on its own, but it can exaggerate the edema which occurs when some other precipitating factor is present. Overtransfusion with saline is an important example; this has been implicated in the edema of the adult respiratory distress syndrome. Another example is the hypoproteinemia of the nephrotic syndrome.

Unknown Etiology

This includes several forms of pulmonary edema. High altitude pulmonary edema is a puzzling condition which occasionally affects climbers and skiers (Figure 6.4). The wedge pressure is normal, so a raised pulmonary venous pressure is unlikely. However, the pulmonary artery pressure is high because of hypoxic vasoconstriction.[†] One hypothesis is that the arteriolar constriction is uneven and that regions of the capillary bed which are therefore not protected from the high pressure tend to leak. There is also evidence of increased permeability, possibly caused by the high capillary pressure or flow in the unprotected regions. Treatment is by descent to a lower altitude. Oxygen should be given if this is available.

Heroin overdosage can cause pulmonary edema. The complication

* See J. B. West: *Respiratory Physiology—The Essentials*, ed. 3, p. 33. Baltimore, Williams & Wilkins, 1985.
[†] See J. B. West: *Respiratory Physiology—The Essentials*, ed. 3, p. 43. Baltimore, Williams & Wilkins, 1985.

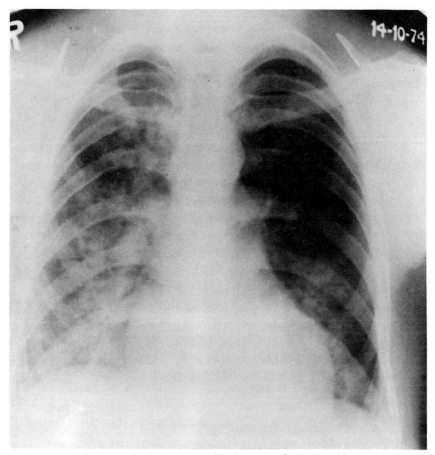

Figure 6.4. Radiograph of a patient with pulmonary edema caused by high altitude. Note the blotchy shadowing, especially on the right side.

is particularly seen in addicts who inject the drug intravenously when it is mixed with various diluents. These might be partly responsible; however, edema can also follow oral ingestion.

Neurogenic pulmonary edema is seen following injuries to the central nervous system, for example, head trauma. The mechanism is unknown, though heightened activity of the sympathetic nervous system has been implicated.

Clinical Features

These depend to some extent on the etiology of the edema, but some generalizations can be made. Dyspnea is usually a prominent symptom;

breathing is typically rapid and shallow. Mild edema may cause few symptoms at rest, but exertional dyspnea is inevitable. Orthopnea (increased dyspnea while recumbent) is common. Paroxysmal nocturnal dyspnea (patient awakes at night with severe dyspnea and wheezing) and Cheyne-Stokes respiration may occur. Cough is frequent and is dry in the early stages. However, in fulminant edema the patient may cough up quantities of pink foaming sputum. Cyanosis may be present.

On auscultation, fine crepitations on inspiration are heard at the lung bases in early edema. In more severe cases, musical rhonchi may be heard. Abnormal heart sounds or murmurs are often present in cardiogenic edema.

The chest radiograph often shows an enlarged heart and prominent pulmonary vessels. Interstitial edema causes Kerley B lines to appear on the radiograph. These are short linear, horizontal markings originating near the pleural surface in the lower zones and caused by edematous interlobular septa. In more severe edema, blotchy shadowing occurs (Figure 6.4). Occasionally this radiates from the hilar regions, giving a so-called bat's-wing or butterfly appearance. The explanation of this distribution is not clear but may be related to the perivascular and peribronchial cuffing which is particularly noticeable around the large vessels in the hilar region (Figures 6.1 and 6.2).

Pulmonary Function

Extensive pulmonary function tests are seldom carried out on patients with pulmonary edema because they are so sick. The most important abnormalities are in the areas of mechanics and gas exchange.

Mechanics

Pulmonary edema reduces the distensibility of the lung and moves the pressure-volume curve downward and to the right (compare Figure 3.1). An important factor in this is the alveolar flooding, which causes a reduction in volume of the affected lung units as a result of surface tension forces and reduces their participation in the pressure-volume curve. In addition, interstitial edema per se probably stiffens the lung by interfering with its elastic properties, though it is difficult to obtain clear evidence on this. Edematous lungs require abnormally large expanding pressures during assisted ventilation and tend to collapse to abnormally small volumes when not actively inflated (Chapter 10).

Airway resistance is typically increased, especially if some of the larger airways contain edema fluid. Reflex bronchoconstriction following stimulation of irritant receptors in the bronchial walls may also play a role. It is possible that in the absence of alveolar edema, interstitial edema increases the resistance of small airways as a result of their peribronchial cuff (Figure 6.1). This can be thought of as actually compressing the small airway or, at least, isolating it from the normal traction of the surrounding parenchyma (Figure 6.5). There is some evidence that this mechanism increases the closing volume (Figure 1.10) and thus predisposes to intermittent ventilation of dependent lung.

Gas Exchange

Interstitial edema has little effect on pulmonary gas exchange. Sometimes a reduced diffusing capacity has been attributed to edematous thickening of the blood-gas barrier, but the evidence is meager. It is possible that cuffs of interstitial edema around small airways (Figures 6.1 and 6.5) can cause intermittent ventilation of dependent regions of the lung leading to hypoxemia, but the importance of this in practice is uncertain.

Alveolar edema causes hypoxemia, chiefly because of blood flow to

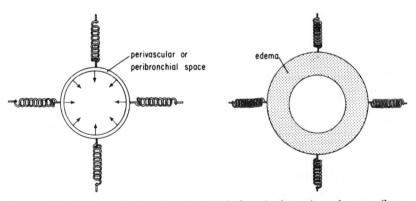

Figure 6.5.   Diagram showing how interstitial edema in the perivascular or peribronchial region can reduce the caliber of the vessel or airway. The cuff isolates the structure from the traction of the surrounding parenchyma.

unventilated units (Figure 10.4). These may be edema-filled alveoli or units supplied by airways that are completely obstructed by fluid. Hypoxic vasoconstriction tends to reduce the true shunt, but often this is large, as much as 50% or more of the total pulmonary blood flow in severe edema. Assisted ventilation with positive end-expiratory pressure (PEEP) often substantially reduces the amount shunt chiefly by clearing edema fluid from some of the larger airways (Figure 10.4).

Lung units with low ventilation-perfusion ratios also contribute to the hypoxemia. These presumably either lie behind airways partly obstructed by edema fluid or are units whose ventilation is reduced by their proximity to edematous alveoli. Such lung units are particularly liable to collapse during treatment with enriched oxygen mixtures (Figures 9.6 and 9.7), but oxygen therapy is often essential to relieve the hypoxemia. A factor which often aggravates the hypoxemia caused by edema following acute myocardial infarction is a low cardiac output, which reduces the P_{O_2} in mixed venous blood.

The alveolar PCO_2 is often normal or low in pulmonary edema because of increased ventilation to the nonedematous alveoli. This is provoked in part by the arterial hypoxemia and also possibly by stimulation of lung receptors (see below). However, in fulminating pulmonary edema, carbon dioxide retention and respiratory acidosis may develop.

Control of Ventilation

Patients with pulmonary edema typically have rapid, shallow breathing. This may be caused by stimulation of J receptors in the alveolar walls and perhaps other vagal afferents. The rapid breathing pattern minimizes the abnormally high elastic work of breathing. Arterial hypoxemia is an additional stimulus to breathing.

Pulmonary Circulation

Pulmonary vascular resistance rises, and hypoxic vasoconstriction of poorly or unventilated areas is one mechanism for this. In addition, perivascular cuffing probably increases the resistance of the extraalveolar vessels (Figures 6.2 and 6.5). Other possible factors are the partial collapse of edematous alveoli, and alveolar wall edema which may compress or distort capillaries.

The topographical distribution of blood flow is sometimes altered by interstitial edema. The normal apex-to-base gradient becomes inverted, with the result that apical flow exceeds basal (Figure 6.6). This is most commonly seen in patients with mitral stenosis. The cause is not fully understood, but it is possible that perivascular cuffs particularly increase the resistance of the lower zone vessels because the lung is less well expanded there (Figure 3.5).

PULMONARY EMBOLISM

This important condition is often preventable and potentially fatal. Small emboli are very common and are frequently undiagnosed.

Pathogenesis

Most pulmonary emboli arise as detached portions of venous thrombi which have formed in the deep veins of the lower extremities. Other sites include the right side of the heart and the pelvic area. Nonthrombotic emboli such as fat, air, and amniotic fluid also occur but are relatively uncommon.

Factors which favor the formation of venous thrombi are:

1. Stasis of blood
2. Alterations in the blood coagulation system
3. Abnormalities of the vessel wall

Stasis of blood is promoted by immobilization following a fracture or an operation, local pressure, or venous obstruction. It is common

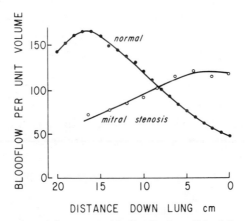

Figure 6.6. Inversion of the topographic distribution of blood flow in a patient with mitral stenosis. The cause is not certain, but interstitial cuffs of edema around the lower zone vessels (Figures 6.2 and 6.5) may be partly responsible.

in congestive heart failure, shock, hypovolemia, dehydration, and varicose veins. An enlarged fibrillating right atrium often contains thrombosed blood.

The intravascular *coagulability of blood* is increased in several conditions such as polycythemia vera and sickle cell disease where the viscosity of the blood increases, thus favoring sluggish flow next to the vessel wall. In other conditions, the mechanism of increased coagulability is poorly understood. Such conditions include malignant diseases, pregnancy, recent trauma, and the use of oral contraceptives. There is no reliable test of an increased tendency for intravascular coagulation, although the prothrombin time and partial thromboplastin time in these conditions are often less than in controls.

The *vessel wall may be damaged* by local trauma or by inflammation. Where there is marked local phlebitis with tenderness, redness, warmth, and swelling, the clot may be more securely adherent to the wall.

The presence of thrombosis in the deep veins of the legs or pelvis is often unsuspected until embolism occurs. Sometimes there is swelling of the limb or local tenderness, and there may be signs of inflammation. Acute dorsiflexion of the ankle may elicit calf pain. Ancillary tests such as venography and the local uptake of radioactive fibrinogen may provide confirmation. Heparin given in small doses reduces the incidence of embolism in patients with deep vein thrombosis.

When the thrombus fragment is released, it is rapidly swept into one of the pulmonary arteries. Very large thrombi impact in a large artery. However, the thrombus may break up and block several smaller vessels. The lower lobes are frequently involved because they have a high blood flow (Figure 3.5).

Pulmonary infarction, that is, death of the embolized tissue, occurs infrequently. More often there is distal hemorrhage and atelectasis, but the alveolar structures remain viable. Infarction is more likely if the embolus completely blocks a large artery or if there is pre-existing lung disease. Infarction results in alveolar filling with extravasated red cells and inflammatory cells and causes an opacity on the radiograph. Occasionally the infarct becomes infected, leading to an abscess. The infrequency of infarction can be explained in part by the fact that most emboli do not completely obstruct the vessel. In addition, bronchial artery anastomoses and the airways supply oxygen to the lung parenchyma.

Clinical Features

The presentation depends considerably on the size of the embolus.

Medium-Sized Emboli

These often present with pleuritic pain accompanied by dyspnea, slight fever, and cough productive of blood-streaked sputum. On ausculation, tachycardia is common and there may be a pleural friction rub. A small pleural effusion may develop. Embolism may mimic pneumonia, and recognition depends on being aware of the diagnosis. The chest radiograph is usually normal; a peripheral wedge-shaped shadow suggests infarction. A lung scan made after injecting radioactive albumin aggregates into the venous circulation shows one or more areas of reduced perfusion (Figure 6.7). The distribution of ventilation, measured with radioactive xenon, is typically normal unless there is pre-existing lung disease.

Massive Emboli

These may produce sudden collapse of the patient with shock, pallor, central chest pain, and sometimes loss of consciousness. The pulse is rapid and weak, the blood pressure is low, and the neck veins are engorged. The electrocardiogram may show the pattern of right ventricular strain. The prognosis is variable, but some 30% of massive emboli prove fatal.

Small Emboli

These are frequently unrecognized. However, repeated small emboli gradually reduce the pulmonary capillary bed, resulting in pulmonary hypertension. There is prominent dyspnea on exercise and this may lead to syncope. On examination a right ventricular heave can be felt, and a loud pulmonary second sound is heard. The ECG and chest radiograph confirm right ventricular hypertrophy.

Pulmonary Function

Pulmonary Circulation

This normally has a large reserve capacity because many capillaries are unfilled. When the pulmonary artery pressure rises, for example, on exercise, these capillaries are recruited and, in addition, some capillary distention occurs.* This reserve means that at least half of

* See J. B. West: *Respiratory Physiology—The Essentials*, ed. 3, p. 36. Baltimore, Williams & Wilkins, 1985.

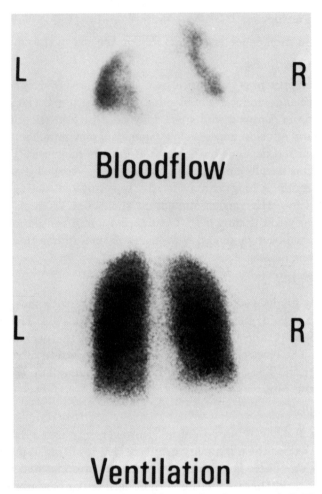

Figure 6.7. Lung scan in a patient with multiple pulmonary emboli. The perfusion image (made with technetium-99m albumin) shows areas of absent bloodflow in both lungs. The ventilation image (made with xenon-133) shows a normal pattern.

the pulmonary circulation can be obstructed by an embolus before there is a substantial rise in pulmonary artery pressure.

In addition to the purely mechanical effects of the embolus, there is some evidence that active vasoconstriction occurs, at least for some minutes after embolization (Figure 6.8). The mechanism is not understood, but in experimental animals, local release of serotonin from

VASCULAR DISEASES

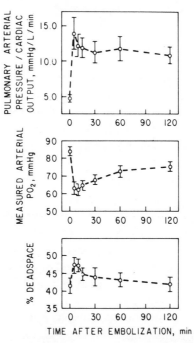

Figure 6.8. Transient changes in pulmonary artery pressure (related to cardiac output), arterial P_{O_2}, and physiologic dead space in dogs following experimental thromboembolism. These suggest active responses of the pulmonary circulation and airways. The importance of these mechanisms in man is unknown. (From D. R. Dantzker, P. D. Wagner, V. W. Tornabene, N. P. Alzaraki, and J. B. West: Gas exchange after pulmonary thromboembolism in dogs. *Circ. Res.* 42:92–103, 1978 (35).)

platelets associated with the embolus has been implicated, as well as reflex vasoconstriction via the sympathetic nervous system. It is not known to what extent these factors operate in man.

If the embolus is large and the pulmonary artery pressure rises considerably, the right ventricle may begin to fail. The end-diastolic pressure increases, arrythmias may develop, and the tricuspid valve may become incompetent. In a few cases pulmonary edema has been seen. This is presumably caused by leakage from those capillaries not protected from the raised pulmonary artery pressure (compare high altitude pulmonary edema).

The increase in pulmonary artery pressure gradually subsides over the subsequent days as the embolus resolves. This occurs both through fibrinolysis and also organization of the clot into a small fibrous scar attached to the vessel wall. Patency of the vessel is thus usually restored.

Mechanics

When a pulmonary artery is occluded by a catheter in man and experimental animals, the ventilation to that area of lung is reduced (34). The mechanism appears to be a direct effect of the reduced alveolar P_{CO_2} on the smooth muscle of the local small airways, causing bronchoconstriction. It can be reversed by adding carbon dioxide to the inspired gas.

Although this airway response to vascular obstruction is generally much weaker than the corresponding vascular response to airway obstruction (hypoxic vasoconstriction), it serves a similar homeostatic role. The reduction in airflow to the unperfused lung reduces the amount of wasted ventilation and thus the physiological dead space. This mechanism is apparently short-lived or not very effective following pulmonary thromboembolism in man, because most measurements of the distribution of ventilation with radioactive xenon made some hours after the episode show no defect in the embolized area. However, in experimental animals transient changes in alveolar P_{O_2}, physiological dead space, and airway resistance often occur following thromboembolism (Figure 6.8) (35).

The elastic properties of the embolized region may change some hours after the event. In experimental animals, ligation of one pulmonary artery is followed by patchy hemorrhagic edema and atelectasis in the affected lung within 24 hr. This has been attributed to loss of pulmonary surfactant, which has a rapid turnover and apparently cannot be replenished in a lung which has lost its pulmonary bloodflow. Again, it is not yet clear how often this occurs in human pulmonary thromboembolism or whether it is part of the pathological process which has been traditionally called infarction. The fact that most emboli do not completely block the vessel presumably limits its occurrence.

Gas Exchange

Moderate hypoxemia without carbon dioxide retention is often seen following pulmonary embolism. Both the physiological shunt and dead space are increased. Various explanations for the hypoxemia have been advanced, including diffusion impairment in areas with high flows and therefore reduced transit time (Figure 2.6), opening up of latent pulmonary artery-vein anastomoses as a consequence of the high pulmonary artery pressure, and blood flow through infarcted areas.

Measurements by the multiple inert gas elimination technique show that the hypoxemia can be explained by ventilation-perfusion inequality (36). Figure 6.9 shows distributions from two patients after massive pulmonary embolism. The most striking features are the large shunts (blood flow to unventilated alveoli) of 20% and 39% and the existence of lung units with very high ventilation-perfusion ratios. The latter can be explained by the embolized regions where the blood flow is typically greatly reduced but not completely abolished. The precise mechanism of the shunts is not certain, but it may be blood flow through areas of hemorrhagic atelectasis.

Occasionally patients with pulmonary embolism also show blood flow to poorly ventilated lung units. It is of interest that in experimental thromboembolism in dogs, no shunt is typically seen, but the hypoxemia can be explained by the increased blood flow through the nonembolized areas of lung. This results in regions with low ventilation-perfusion ratios which depress the alveolar P_{O_2}. It is not clear how often this pattern occurs in human disease, but it is difficult to make many measurements in these patients because they are usually very ill.

The arterial P_{CO_2} following pulmonary embolism is maintained at the normal level by increasing the ventilation to the alveoli. The increase in ventilation may be substantial because of the large physiological dead space, and therefore wasted ventilation, caused by the embolized areas.

Some investigators have suggested that the difference in P_{CO_2} between arterial blood and end-tidal gas is a useful test for pulmonary embolism. The mixed alveolar P_{CO_2} tends to be low because of the high $\dot{V}_A/\dot{Q}$ in the embolized region, and since there is little uneven ventilation in this disease, the end-tidal P_{CO_2} is a useful measure of the mixed alveolar value.

In practice, this test is less sensitive than originally anticipated for two reasons. First, many emboli do not cause complete occlusion of

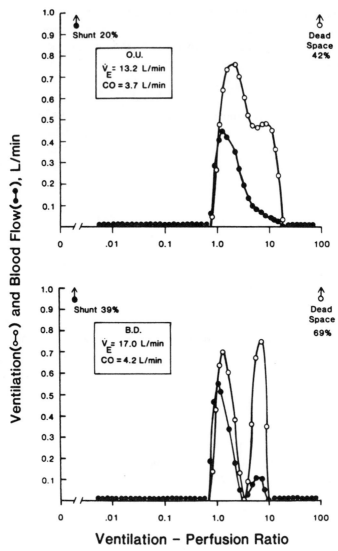

Figure 6.9. Distributions of ventilation-perfusion ratios in two patients with acute massive pulmonary embolism. Note that in both instances, the hypoxemia could be explained by large shunts. In addition, there was a large increase in ventilation to lung units with abnormally high ventilation-perfusion ratios representing the embolized regions. (From G. E. D'Alonzo, J. S. Bower, P. DeHart, and D. R. Dantzker: The mechanisms of abnormal gas exchange in acute massive pulmonary embolism. *Am. Rev. Respir. Dis.* 128:170–172, 1983 (36).)

the vessel, with the result that the P_{CO_2} in the affected region is not reduced to very low levels. Second, insofar as the embolized areas are poorly ventilated because of local bronchoconstriction, their contribution to end-tidal gas is reduced.

PULMONARY HYPERTENSION

The normal mean pulmonary artery pressure is about 15 mm Hg; an increased level is called pulmonary hypertension. There are three principal mechanisms of this.

1. Increase in Left Atrial Pressure. Examples are mitral stenosis or left ventricular failure. This is sometimes called passive pulmonary hypertension, since the changes in pulmonary artery pressure are led by those in the left atrium. However, sustained increases in left atrial pressure lead to structured changes in the walls of the small pulmonary arteries, including medial hypertrophy and intimal thickening. Clinically an increase in left atrial pressure can cause dyspnea, hemoptysis, and pulmonary edema.

2. Increase in Pulmonary Blood Flow. This occurs in congenital heart disease with left-to-right shunts through ventricular or atrial septal defects or a patent ductus arteriosus. Initially the rise in pulmonary artery pressure is relatively small because of the ability of the pulmonary capillaries to accommodate high flows by recruitment and distension. However, sustained high flows result in histologic changes in the walls of the small arteries, and eventually the pulmonary artery pressures may reach systemic levels, causing some right-to-left shunting and arterial hypoxemia.

3. Increase in Pulmonary Vascular Resistance. This is the commonest cause of severe pulmonary hypertension. Again, three categories can be described.

a. Vasoconstrictive, principally because of alveolar hypoxia as occurs at high altitude. This is also a component in the hypertension of chronic bronchitis and emphysema. Serotonin may cause transient vasoconstriction following thromboembolism, and the release of catecholamines may be a factor in some conditions.

b. Obstructive, as in thromboembolism. In addition the vessels may be occluded by circulating fat, air, amniotic fluid, or cancer cells. In schistosomiasis, the parasites lodge in small arteries causing a marked reaction.

c. Obliterative, as in emphysema where the capillary bed is partly destroyed (Figures 4.2 and 4.3). Various forms of arteritis can also occur such as in polyarteritis nodosa. Rarely, the small veins are involved as in pulmonary veno-occlusive disease.

Primary Pulmonary Hypertension

This is an uncommon disorder of unknown cause; some cases may be due to unrecognized, repeated small emboli. The majority of patients are females in the age range 20–40 years. Histological examination of the lung shows an increase in smooth muscle in the small pulmonary arteries.

The chief symptom is dyspnea on exercise. Syncope may occur. Examination reveals signs of right ventricular hypertrophy which are confirmed by the ECG and chest radiographic appearances. Mild hypoxemia may be present but ventilatory tests are usually normal. The disease typically progresses inexorably and death occurs within a few years.

Cor Pulmonale

This term refers to right heart disease secondary to primary disease of the lung. The occurrence of right ventricular hypertrophy and fluid retention in chronic obstructive lung disease was discussed on page 78. The same findings may occur late in restrictive lung disease.

The various factors which lead to pulmonary hypertension include obliteration of the capillary bed by destruction of alveolar walls or interstitial fibrosis, hypoxic vasoconstriction, hypertrophy of smooth muscle in the walls of the small arteries, and increased viscosity of the blood caused by polycythemia. Whether the term "right heart failure" should be applied to all these patients is disputed. In some the output of the heart is increased because it is operating high on the Starling curve, and the output can increase further on exercise. The principal physiological abnormality in these patients is fluid retention. However, in others, true failure develops. Some physicians restrict the term cor pulmonale to those patients who have ECG evidence of right ventricular hypertrophy.

PULMONARY ARTERIOVENOUS FISTULA

This uncommon condition is characterized by an abnormal communication between a pulmonary artery and vein. About half the patients also have telangiectases of the skin or mucous membranes, suggesting that there is a general vascular defect. There is sometimes a family history of telangiectasia.

Small lesions cause no functional disturbances and may be found on a routine chest radiograph. Larger fistulae cause true shunts and hypoxemia. The arterial P_{O_2} is depressed far below the expected value during oxygen breathing (Figure 2.8). Sometimes a bruit can be detected over the fistula by auscultation. Finger clubbing is common.

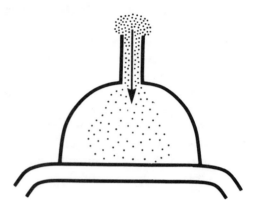

chapter 7

Occupational and Other Diseases

DISEASES CAUSED BY INHALED PARTICLES

Many occupational or industrial lung diseases are caused by inhaled dusts. Atmospheric pollutants are also important factors in the etiology of other diseases such as chronic bronchitis, emphysema, and bronchial carcinoma, so we shall start by looking at the environment that we all live in.

Atmospheric Pollutants

Carbon Monoxide

This is the largest pollutant by weight in the United States (Figure 7.1, *left*). It is produced by the incomplete combustion of carbon in fuels, chiefly in the automobile engine (Figure 7.1, *right*). The main hazard of carbon monoxide is its propensity to tie up hemoglobin; because carbon monoxide has over 200 times the affinity of oxygen, it

Atmospheric pollutants

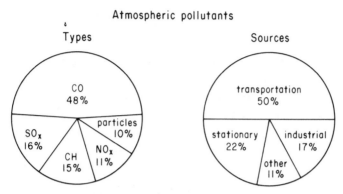

Types   Sources

Figure 7.1. Air pollutants (by weight) in the United States, 1974. Note that transportation sources, especially automobiles, account for the largest amount of pollutants. Stationary sources, particularly power stations, account for 22%. (SO_x, sulfur oxides; NO_x, nitrogen oxides; CH, hydrocarbons.) (From the Environmental Protection Agency.)

competes very successfully with this gas.* A commuter using a busy urban freeway may have 5–10% of his hemoglobin bound to carbon monoxide, particularly if he is a cigarette smoker, and there is evidence that this can impair mental skills. The emission of carbon monoxide and other pollutants by automobile engines can be reduced by installing a catalytic converter which processes the exhaust gases.

Sulfur Oxides

These are corrosive, poisonous gases produced when sulfur-containing fuels are burnt, chiefly by power stations. These gases cause inflammation of the mucous membranes, eyes, upper respiratory tract, and bronchial mucosa. Short-term exposure to high concentrations causes pulmonary edema. Long-term exposure to lower levels results in chronic bronchitis in experimental animals. The best way to reduce emissions of sulfur oxides is to use low-sulfur fuels, but these are more expensive.

Hydrocarbons

Hydrocarbons, like carbon monoxide, represent unburned wasted fuel. They are not toxic at concentrations normally found in the atmos-

* See J. B. West: *Respiratory Physiology—The Essentials*, ed. 3, p. 72. Baltimore, Williams & Wilkins, 1985.

phere. However, they are hazardous because they form photochemical oxidants under the influence of sunlight.

Particulate Matter

This includes particles with a wide range of sizes up to visible smoke and soot. Major sources are power stations and industrial plants. Often their emission can be reduced by processing the waste air stream by filtering or scrubbing, although removing the smallest particles is often expensive.

Nitrogen Oxides

These are produced when fossil fuels (coal, oil) are burned at very high temperatures in power stations and automobiles. These gases cause inflammation of the eyes and upper respiratory tract during smoggy conditions. At higher concentrations they can cause acute tracheitis, acute bronchitis, and pulmonary edema. The yellow haze of smog is due to these gases.

Photochemical Oxidants

These include ozone and other substances such as peroxyacyl nitrates, aldehydes, and acrolein. They are not primary emissions but are produced by the action of sunlight on hydrocarbons and nitrogen oxides. They cause inflammation of the eyes and respiratory tract, damage to vegetation, and offensive odors. In higher concentrations, ozone causes pulmonary edema. These oxidants contribute to the thick haze of smog.

The concentration of atmospheric pollutants is often greatly increased by a temperature inversion, that is, a low layer of cold air beneath warmer air. This prevents the normal escape of warm surface air with its pollutants to the upper atmosphere. The deleterious effects of a temperature inversion are particularly marked in a low lying area surrounded by hills, such as the Los Angeles basin.

Cigarette Smoke

This is one of the most important pollutants in practice because it is inhaled by devotees in concentrations many times greater than those in the atmosphere. It includes about 4% carbon monoxide, enough to raise the carboxyhemoglobin level in a smoker's blood to 10%, which is sufficient to impair exercise and mental performance. The smoke also contains the alkaloid nicotine, which stimulates the autonomic nervous system, causing tachycardia, hypertension, and sweating. Aromatic hydrocarbons and other substances, loosely called "tars," are apparently responsible for the high risk of bronchial carcinoma in cigarette smokers—40 times that of nonsmokers in males smoking 35 cigarettes/day. Increased risks of chronic bronchitis and emphysema and of coronary heart disease are also well documented. A single cigarette causes a marked increase in airway resistance in many smokers and nonsmokers (Figure 3.2).

Deposition of Aerosols in the Lung

The term "aerosol" refers to a collection of particles which remains airborne for a substantial amount of time. Many pollutants exist in this form, and their pattern of deposition in the lung depends chiefly on their size. The properties of aerosols are also important in understanding the action of inhaled bronchodilators. Three mechanisms of deposition are recognized (37).

Impaction

Impaction refers to the tendency of the largest inspired particles to fail to turn the corners of the respiratory tract. As a result, many particles impinge on the mucous surfaces of the nose and pharynx (Figure 7.2A) and also on the bifurcations of the large airways. Once a particle strikes the wet surface it is trapped and not subsequently released into the gas. The nose is remarkably efficient at removing the largest particles by this mechanism; almost all particles greater than 20 μ in diameter and about 95% of particles of 5 μ in diameter are filtered by the nose during resting breathing. Figure 7.3 shows that most of the deposition of particles over 3 μ in diameter occurs in the nasopharynx during nose breathing.

Sedimentation

Sedimentation is the gradual settling of particles due to their weight (Figure 7.2B). It is particularly important for medium-sized particles (1–5 μ) because the larger particles are removed by impaction and the smaller particles settle so slowly. Deposition by sedimentation occurs extensively in the small airways, including the terminal and respiratory bronchioles. The chief reason is simply that the dimensions of those airways are very small and therefore the particles have a shorter

Particle deposition

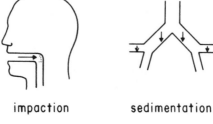

Mechanism :	impaction	sedimentation	diffusion
Particle size :	large (>5μ)	medium (1−5μ)	small (<0.1μ)
Representative site :	nasopharynx	small airways	alveoli

| A | B | C |

Figure 7.2.   Scheme of deposition of aerosols in the lung. The "representative sites" shown do not mean that the mechanism does not operate elsewhere. For example, impaction also occurs in the medium-sized bronchi and diffusion also occurs in the large and small airways. (See text for details.)

distance to fall. Note that the particles, unlike gases, are not able to diffuse from the respiratory bronchioles to the alveoli because of their negligibly small diffusion rate.*

Figure 7.4 shows accumulations of dust around the terminal and respiratory bronchioles of a coal miner with early pneumoconiosis (38). While the retention of dust depends on both deposition and clearance, and it is likely that some of this dust was transported from peripheral alveoli, the appearance is a graphic reminder of the vulnerability of this region of the lung. It has been suggested that some of the earliest changes in chronic bronchitis and emphysema are secondary to the deposition of atmospheric pollutants (including tobacco smoke particles) in these small airways.

Diffusion

Diffusion is the random movement of particles as a result of their continuous bombardment by gas molecules (Figure 7.2C). It occurs to a significant extent only in the smallest particles less than 0.1 μ in

* See J. B. West: *Respiratory Physiology—The Essentials*, ed. 3, p. 6. Baltimore, Williams & Wilkins, 1985.

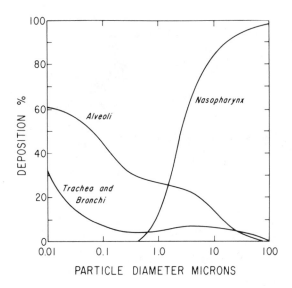

PARTICLE DIAMETER MICRONS

Figure 7.3. Site of deposition of aerosols. Note that the largest particles remain in the nasopharynx, but the very small particles can penetrate to the alveoli. (Modified from M. Newhouse, J. Sanchis, and J. Bienenstock: Lung defense mechanisms. *N. Engl. J. Med.* 295:990–998, 1045–1052, 1976 (37).)

diameter. Deposition by diffusion chiefly takes place in the small airways and alveoli where the distances to the wall are least. However, some deposition by this mechanism also occurs in the larger airways.

It should be noted that many inhaled particles are not deposited at all but are exhaled with the next breath. In fact, only some 30% of 0.5 μ particles may be left in the lung during normal resting breathing. These particles are too small to impact or sediment to a large extent. In addition, they are too large to diffuse significantly. As a result, they do not move from the terminal and respiratory bronchioles to the alveoli by diffusion, the normal mode of gas movement in this region. It should also be pointed out that small particles may become larger during inspiration by aggregation or absorbing water.

The pattern of ventilation affects the amount of aerosol deposition. Slow, deep breaths increase the penetration into the lung and thus the amount of dust deposited by sedimentation and diffusion. Exercise results in higher rates of airflow and particularly increases deposition by impaction. In general, deposition of dust is proportional to the ventilation during exercise, which is therefore an important factor during work at the coal face.

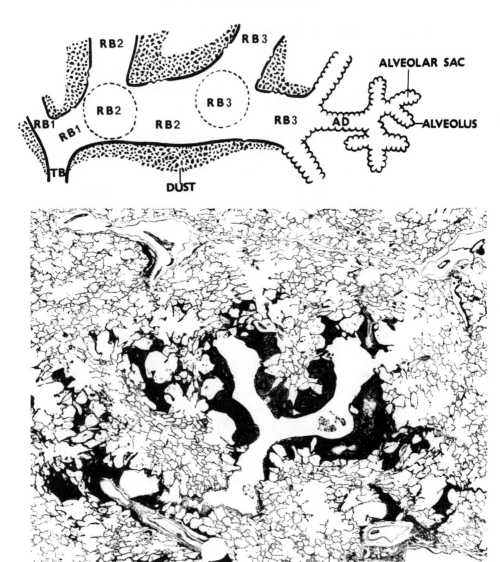

Figure 7.4. Section of lung from a coal miner showing accumulations of dust around the respiratory bronchioles. These small airways show some dilatation, sometimes called focal emphysema. (From A. G. Heppleston and J. G. Leopold: Chronic pulmonary emphysema: anatomy and pathogenesis. *Am. J. Med.* 31:279–291, 1961 (38).)

Clearance of Deposited Particles

Fortunately the lung is very efficient at removing particles which are deposited within it. Two distinct clearance mechanisms exist: the mucociliary system and the alveolar macrophages (Figure 7.5).

Mucociliary System

Mucus is produced by two sources: 1) Bronchial seromucous glands situated deep in the bronchial walls (Figures 4.6, 4.7, and 4.13). Both mucus-producing and serous-producing cells are present, and ducts lead the mucus to the airway surface. 2) Goblet cells which form part of the bronchial epithelium.

The normal mucous film is about 5–10 μ thick and has two layers (Figure 7.6). The superficial gel layer is relatively tenacious and

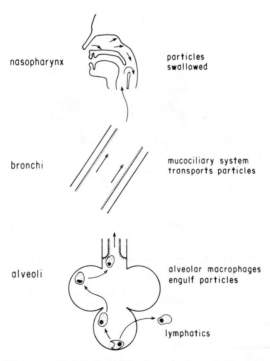

nasopharynx   particles swallowed

bronchi   mucociliary system transports particles

alveoli   alveolar macrophages engulf particles

lymphatics

Figure 7.5. Clearance of inhaled particles from the lung. Particles which deposit on the surface of the airways are transported by the mucociliary escalator and swallowed. Particles which reach the alveoli are engulfed by macrophages, which either migrate to the ciliary surface or escape via the lymphatics.

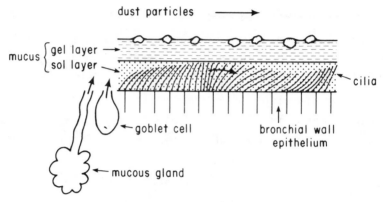

Figure 7.6. Mucociliary escalator. The mucous film consists of a superficial gel layer which traps inhaled particles and a deeper sol layer. It is propelled by cilia.

viscous. As a result, it is efficient at trapping deposited particles. The deeper sol layer is less viscous and thus allows the cilia to beat within it easily. It is likely that the abnormal retention of secretions that occurs in some diseases is caused by changes in the composition of the mucus, with the result that it cannot be easily propelled by the cilia.

The mucus contains the immunoglobulin IgA, which is derived from plasma cells and lymphoid tissue. This humoral factor is an important defense against foreign proteins, bacteria, and viruses.

The cilia are 5–7 μ in length and beat in a synchronized fashion at between 1000 and 1500 times/min. During the forward stroke the tips of the cilia apparently come in contact with the gel layer, thus propelling it, but during the recovery phase, the cilia are bent so much that they move entirely within the sol layer where the resistance is less.

The mucous blanket moves up at about 1 mm/min in small peripheral airways but as fast as 2 cm/min in the trachea, and eventually the particles reach the level of the pharynx where they are swallowed. The clearance of a healthy bronchial mucosa is essentially complete in less than 24 hr. In very dusty environments mucous secretion may be increased so much that cough and expectoration assist in the clearance.

The normal operation of the mucociliary system is affected by pollution or disease. The cilia can apparently be paralyzed by the inhalation of toxic gases such as oxides of sulfur and nitrogen and perhaps by tobacco smoke. In acute inflammation of the respiratory tract the bronchial epithelium may be denuded. Changes in the character of the mucus may occur with infection, thus making it difficult for the cilia to transport it. Mucous plugging of bronchi occurs in asthma but the mechanism is unknown. Finally, in chronic infections such as bronchiectasis or chronic bronchitis, the volume of secretions may be so great that they overload the ciliary transport system.

Alveolar Macrophages

The mucociliary system stops short of the alveoli and particles deposited there are engulfed by macrophages. These amoeboid cells roam around the surface of the alveoli. When they swallow foreign particles, either they migrate to the small airways where they load on to the mucociliary escalator (Figure 7.5) or they leave the lung in the lymphatics or possibly the blood. When the dust burden is very large or the dust particles are toxic, some of the macrophages migrate through the walls of the respiratory bronchioles and dump their dust there. Figure 7.4 shows accumulations of dust around the respiratory bronchioles in the lung of a coal miner. If the dust is toxic, such as silica, a fibrous reaction is stimulated in this region.

The macrophages not only transport bacteria out of the lung but also kill them in situ by means of the lysozymes they contain. As a consequence, the alveoli very quickly become sterile, although it takes some time for the dead organisms to be cleared from the lung. Immunological mechanisms are also presumably important in the antibacterial action of macrophages.

Normal macrophage activity can be impaired by various factors such as cigarette smoke, oxidant gases such as ozone, alveolar hypoxia, radiation, the administration of corticosteroids, and the ingestion of alcohol. Macrophages which engulf particles of silica are often destroyed by this toxic material.

Coal Workers' Pneumoconiosis

The term "pneumoconiosis" refers to parenchymal lung disease caused by inorganic dust inhalation. The commonest is that seen in coal workers, and it is directly related to the amount of coal dust to which the miner has been exposed.

Pathology

Early and late forms of the disease should be distinguished. In simple pneumoconiosis there are aggregations of coal particles around terminal and respiratory bronchioles, with some dilatation of these small airways (Figure 7.4). In the advanced form of the disease, known as progressive massive fibrosis, condensed masses of black fibrous tissue infiltrated with dust are seen. Not all miners exposed to heavy dust concentrations develop progressive massive fibrosis.

Clinical Features

Simple pneumoconiosis apparently causes little disability in spite of its radiographic appearances. The dyspnea and cough which often accompany the disease are closely related to the smoking history of the miner and are probably chiefly caused by associated chronic bronchitis and emphysema. Often the miners' working conditions are poor and conducive to chronic obstructive lung disease. By contrast, progressive massive fibrosis usually causes increasing dyspnea and may terminate in respiratory failure.

The chest radiograph of simple pneumoconiosis shows a delicate micronodular mottling, and various stages in the advance of the disease are recognized depending on the density of the shadows. Progressive massive fibrosis results in large irregular dense opacities often surrounded by abnormally radiolucent lung. Figure 7.7 shows an unusual example in which simple pulmonary function tests were within normal limits in spite of the striking amount of lung disease (39).

Pulmonary Function

Simple pneumoconiosis usually causes little functional impairment by itself. However, sometimes a small reduction in forced expiratory volume, a rise in residual volume, and a fall in arterial P_{O_2} are seen. It is often difficult to know whether these changes are caused by associated chronic bronchitis and emphysema.

Progressive massive fibrosis causes a mixed obstructive and restrictive pattern. Distortion of the airways results in irreversible obstructive changes, while the large masses of fibrous tissue reduce the useful volume of the lung. Increasing hypoxemia, cor pulmonale, and terminal respiratory failure may occur.

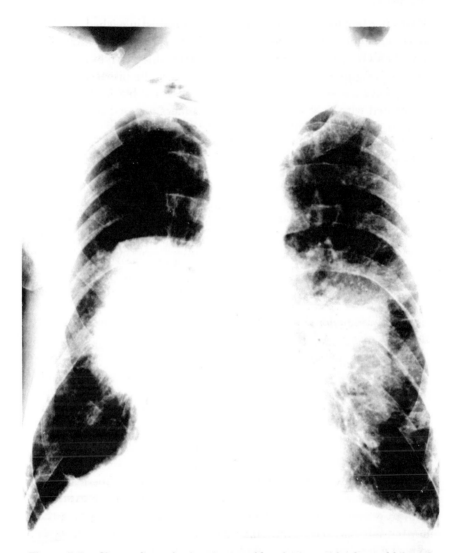

Figure 7.7. Chest radiograph of an 81-year-old coal miner with advanced bilateral progressive massive fibrosis. Astonishingly, simple pulmonary function tests were within normal limits for his age. For example, his arterial P_{O_2} and P_{CO_2} were 79 and 36 mm Hg, respectively. (From W. T. Ulmer and G. Reichel: Functional impairment in coal worker's pneumoconiosis. *Ann. N. Y. Acad. Sci.* 200:405–412, 1972 (39).)

Silicosis

This pneumoconiosis is caused by the inhalation of silica (SiO_2) during quarrying, mining, or sandblasting. Unlike virtually inert coal dust, silica particles are toxic and provoke a marked fibrous reaction in the lung.

Pathology

Silicotic nodules composed of concentric whorls of dense collagen fibers are found around respiratory bronchioles, inside alveoli, and along the lymphatics. Silica particles may be seen in the nodules.

Clinical Features

Mild forms of the disease may cause no symptoms, although the chest radiograph shows fine nodular markings. Advanced disease results in cough and dyspnea, especially on exercise. The radiograph sometimes shows streaks of fibrous tissue and progressive massive fibrosis may develop. The disease may progress long after exposure to the dust has ceased. There is an increased risk of pulmonary tuberculosis.

Pulmonary Function

The changes are similar to those seen in coal workers' pneumoconiosis but are often more severe. In advanced disease, generalized interstitial fibrosis may develop, with a restrictive type of defect, severe dyspnea and hypoxemia on exercise, and a reduced diffusing capacity.

Asbestosis

Asbestos is a naturally occurring fibrous mineral silicate which is used in a variety of industrial applications including heat insulation, pipe lagging, roofing materials, and brake linings. Asbestos fibers are long and thin, and it is possible that their aerodynamic characteristics allow them to penetrate far into the lung. When they are in the lung they may become encased in proteinaceous material. If these are coughed up in the sputum, they are known as asbestos bodies.

Three health hazards are recognized.

1. Diffuse interstitial fibrosis may gradually occur after heavy exposure. There is progressive dyspnea, especially on exercise, weakness, and finger clubbing. On auscultation there are fine basal crepitations. The chest radiograph shows haziness or mottling. Pulmonary function

tests in advanced disease reveal a typical restrictive pattern with reductions of vital capacity and lung compliance. A fall in diffusing capacity occurs relatively early in the disease.

2. Bronchial carcinoma is a common complication. Cigarette smoking is often an aggravating factor.

3. Pleural disease may occur following trivial exposure, for example, in a housewife who washes the clothes of an asbestos worker. Pleural thickening and plaques are common but are usually harmless. Malignant mesothelioma may develop as much as 40 years after light exposure. It causes progressive restriction of chest movement, severe chest pain, and a rapid downhill course.

Other Pneumoconioses

A variety of other dusts cause simple pneumoconiosis. Examples include iron and its oxides, which cause siderosis and result in a striking, mottled radiographic appearance. Antimony and tin are other culprits. Beryllium exposure results in granulomatous lesions of acute or chronic types. The latter results in interstitial fibrosis with its typical restrictive pattern of dysfunction. The disease is now much less common than it was following strict control of beryllium in industry.

Byssinosis

Some inhaled dusts cause airway rather than alveolar reactions. A good example is byssinosis, which follows exposure to cotton dust, especially in the cardroom where the fibers are initially processed.

The pathogenesis is not fully understood, but it appears that the inhalation of some active component in the bracts (leaves around the stem of the cotton boll) leads to the release of histamine from mast cells in the lung. The resulting bronchoconstriction causes dyspnea and wheezing. A feature of the disease is that the symptoms are worst on entering the mill, especially after a period of absence. For this reason it is sometimes known as "Monday fever." The symptoms include dyspnea, tightness of the chest, wheezing, and an irritating cough. Workers with previous chronic bronchitis or asthma are especially susceptible.

Pulmonary function tests shown an obstructive pattern with reductions in $FEV_{1.0}$ FEV/FVC%, $FEF_{25-75\%}$, and VC. Airway resistance measured in a body plethysmograph is increased. In addition, the amount of inequality of ventilation as determined by nitrogen washout rises following exposure. Typically these abnormalities gradually become worse over the course of the working day, but partial or complete recovery occurs during the night or over the weekend. There is no evidence of parenchymal involvement and the chest radiograph is normal. However, epidemiological studies show that daily exposure over 20 years or so causes permanent impairment of lung function of the type associated with chronic obstructive lung disease.

Occupational Asthma

Various occupations involve exposure to allergenic organic dusts, and some individuals develop hypersensitivity. These include flour mill workers who are sensitive to the wheat weevil, printers exposed to gum acacia, and workers handling fur or feathers. Toluene diisocyanate (TDI) is a special case because some individuals develop an extreme sensitivity to this substance, which is used in the manufacture of polyurethane products.

MALIGNANT DISEASES

Bronchial Carcinoma

This important disease will only be briefly discussed because its effects on pulmonary function are minor in the context of diagnosis and treatment. The incidence of the disease is awesome; it is the commonest form of malignancy in the male and accounts for 25% of all male cancer deaths. Much of this disease is preventable.

Etiology

There is strong evidence that cigarette smoking is a major factor. Epidemiological studies show that an individual who smokes 20 cigarettes a day has about 20 times the chance of dying from the disease that a nonsmoker of the same age and sex has. Furthermore, the risk decreases dramatically if the individual stops smoking.

   The specific causative agents in cigarette smoke have not been identified, but many potential carcinogenic substances are present, including aromatic hydrocarbons, phenols, and radioisotopes. Many smoke particles are submicronic and penetrate far into the lung. However, the fact that many bronchogenic carcinomas originate in the large bronchi suggests that deposition by impaction or sedimentation may play an important role (Figure 7.2). Also, the large bronchi are exposed to a high concentration of tobacco smoke products as the material is transported from the more peripheral regions by the mucociliary system. Individuals who do not inhale smoke probably have a lower risk, though this is disputed.

Other etiological factors are recognized. Urban dwellers are more at risk, suggesting that atmospheric pollution plays a part. This is hardly surprising in view of the variety of chronic respiratory tract irritants which exist in city air (Figure 7.1). Occupational factors also exist, especially exposure to chromates, nickel, arsenic, asbestos, and radioactive gases.

Pathology

Four main types of primary lung cancer are recognized. 1) Squamous cell. These tend to grow more slowly and metastasize later than other types. 2) Undifferentiated. These may be small cell (oat cell) or large cell in form. They grow fast and the prognosis is especially poor. 3) Adenocarcinomas. These often grow slowly and may remain clinically silent until metastases occur. They are apparently not related to smoking. 4) Alveolar cell carcinomas. These arise from the alveolar epithelium and tend to grow along the alveolar walls. In addition, secondary carcinomas from other organs frequently occur in the lung.

Clinical Features

An unproductive cough or hemoptysis is a common early symptom. Sometimes hoarseness is the first clue, due to involvement of the left recurrent laryngeal nerve. Dyspnea due to pleural effusion or bronchial obstruction, and chest pain caused by pleural involvement are usually late symptoms. Examination of the chest is often negative, though signs of lobar collapse or consolidation may be found. The chest radiograph is often crucial, but a small carcinoma may not be visible. Bronchoscopy and sputum cytology are valuable aids to early diagnosis.

Pulmonary Function

The objective is to diagnose a carcinoma of the bronchus early enough to remove it surgically. Pulmonary function tests are rarely of value in this regard. On the other hand, lung function is often impaired in moderately advanced disease.

A large pleural effusion causes a restrictive defect (page 109), as may the collapse of a lobe following complete bronchial obstruction. Partial obstruction of a large bronchus can result in an obstructive pattern. The obstruction can be due to either a tumor of the bronchial wall or compression by an enlarged lymph gland. The latter is particularly common in the right middle lobe. Sometimes the movement of the lung on the affected side is seen to lag behind the normal lung, and air may cycle back and forth between the normal and obstructed lobes.* This is known as pendelluft (swinging air). Partial or complete bronchial obstruction usually causes some hypoxemia.

INFECTIOUS DISEASES

Again, although these diseases are of great importance in the general context of internal medicine, they do not generally cause specific patterns of impaired function, and pulmonary function tests are of little value in the management of these patients. This section is therefore very brief.

Pneumonia

This term refers to inflammation of the lung parenchyma associated with alveolar filling by exudate.

Pathology

The alveoli are crammed with cells, chiefly polymorphonuclear leucocytes. Resolution may occur, with restoration of the normal morphology. On the other hand, suppuration may result in necrosis of tissue, causing a lung abscess. Special forms of pneumonia include that following aspiration of gastric fluid or animal or mineral oil (lipoid pneumonia). Psittacosis is a form transmitted from infected parrots by a rickettsia.

Clinical Features

These vary considerably depending on the causative organism, the age of the patient, and his general condition. Usually there is malaise, fever, and cough. Commonly pleuritic pain occurs, worse on deep

---

* See J. B. West: *Respiratory Physiology—The Essentials*, ed. 3, p. 155. Baltimore, Williams & Wilkins, 1985.

breathing. Examination reveals rapid shallow breathing, tachycardia, and sometimes cyanosis. There are often signs of consolidation and the chest radiograph shows opacification. This may involve all of a lobe (lobar pneumonia), but frequently the distribution is patchy (bronchopneumonia). Sputum examination and culture frequently identify the causative organism.

Pulmonary Function

Since the pneumonic region is not ventilated, it causes shunting and hypoxemia. The severity of this depends on the local pulmonary blood flow, which may be substantially reduced either by the disease process itself or hypoxic vasoconstriction. However, patients with severe pneumonia may be cyanosed. Carbon dioxide retention does not generally occur. Chest movement may be restricted by pleural pain or by a pleural effusion.

Tuberculosis

Pulmonary tuberculosis takes many forms. Early lesions do not affect pulmonary function, but in the late stages of the disease severe functional impairment may occur, leading to respiratory failure. Advanced disease is much less common now because of treatment with antituberculous drugs.

The initial infection results in a primary complex with hilar lymph node enlargement. This rapidly resolves and is not generally recognized. The postprimary infection is usually in the apices of the lungs, apparently because the high ventilation-perfusion ratio there and the resulting high P_{O_2} (Figure 3.5) provide a favorable environment for the growth of the bacillus. If this heals, as it generally does, no functional impairment results.

Extension of the infection may cause pneumonia, miliary infection, cavitation, lobar collapse, or pleural effusion. Ultimately, severe fibrosis may develop, with restrictive impairment of function.

Pulmonary Involvement in AIDS

Acquired immunodeficiency syndrome (AIDS) frequently involves the lung. The commonest infection is *Pneumocystis carinii*, but *Mycobacterium avium-intracellulare* and cytomegalovirus infections also occur often. Less frequent infections include tuberculosis and *Legionella*. Kaposi's sarcoma may occur in the lung. In patients from high risk groups who present with these pulmonary problems, AIDS should be suspected.

SUPPURATIVE DISEASES

Bronchiectasis

This disease is characterized by dilatation of bronchi with local suppuration.

Pathology

The mucosal surface of the affected bronchi shows loss of ciliated epithelium, squamous metaplasia and infiltration with inflammatory cells. Pus is present in the lumen during infective exacerbations. The surrounding lung often shows fibrosis and old inflammatory changes.

Clinical Features

The disease usually follows childhood pneumonia, and the prevalence has fallen greatly since the introduction of antibiotics. The cardinal feature is a productive cough with yellow or green sputum. This may occur only after a cold or it may be present continuously. There may be hemoptysis and halitosis. Crepitations are often heard, and finger clubbing is seen in severe cases. The chest radiograph shows increased markings.

Pulmonary Function

Mild disease causes no loss of function. In more advanced cases there is a reduction of FEV and VC because of chronic inflammatory changes including fibrosis. Radioactive gas measurements show reduced ventilation and pulmonary blood flow in the affected area, but there may be a greatly increased bronchial artery supply to the diseased tissue. Hypoxemia may develop as a result of blood flow through unventilated lung.

Cystic Fibrosis

This is a disease of all exocrine glands caused by a genetic abnormality. In the lung it takes the form of bronchiectasis and bronchiolitis.

Pathology

The principal organ affected is the pancreas, where the tissue atrophies and the ducts remain as dilatated cysts. The bronchiectasis results in part from excessive secretions from the hypertrophied mucous glands. Ciliary activity is also apparently impaired, and mucous plugging of small airways and chronic infection follow. Malnutrition secondary to pancreatic failure may lower resistance to infection.

Clinical Features

A few patients die of meconium ileus shortly after birth, and others remain small and malnourished. The respiratory symptoms include productive cough, frequent chest infections and decreased exercise tolerance. Finger clubbing is often prominent. Auscultation may reveal coarse rales and rhonchi. The chest radiograph is abnormal early in the disease and shows areas of consolidation, fibrosis, and cystic changes. In young children, the finding of a high sodium concentration in the sweat confirms the diagnosis.

Until recently, death almost invariably occurred before adulthood, but with improved treatment of chest infections, survival into the 20's is now sometimes seen. Indeed, the disease should be considered when a teenager or a young adult presents with features of chronic bronchitis.

Pulmonary Function

An abnormal distribution of ventilation and an increased alveolar-arterial O_2 difference are early changes. Some investigators report that tests of small airways function, such as flow rates at low lung volumes, may detect minimal disease. There is a decrease in $FEV_{1.0}$ and $FEF_{25-75\%}$ which does not respond to bronchodilators. RV and FRC are raised and there may be loss of elastic recoil. Exercise tolerance falls as the disease progresses.

SECTION THREE
FUNCTION OF THE FAILING LUNG

8. Respiratory failure
9. Oxygen therapy
10. Mechanical ventilation

Respiratory failure is the end result of many types of chronic lung disease. In addition, the condition is increasingly encountered as a complication of severe trauma, septicemia, and other acute conditions. This section is devoted to the physiological principles of respiratory failure and its chief modes of treatment: oxygen administration and mechanical ventilation.

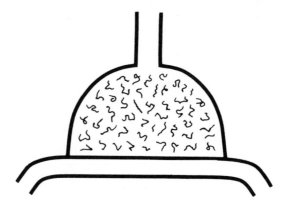

chapter 8

Respiratory Failure

Respiratory failure is said to occur when the lung fails to adequately oxygenate the arterial blood and/or fails to prevent CO_2 retention. There is no absolute definition of the levels of arterial P_{O_2} and P_{CO_2} which indicate respiratory failure. However, as a general guide, a P_{O_2} of less than 60 mm Hg or a P_{CO_2} of more than 50 mm Hg are numbers which are often quoted. In practice the significance of such values depends considerably on the past history of the patient.

GAS EXCHANGE IN RESPIRATORY FAILURE

Patterns of Arterial Blood Gases

Various types of respiratory failure are associated with different degrees of hypoxemia and CO_2 retention. Figure 8.1 shows an O_2-CO_2 diagram with the line for a respiratory exchange ratio of 0.8. Pure hypoventilation leading to respiratory failure moves the arterial P_{O_2} and P_{CO_2} in the direction indicated by the *arrow A* (compare Figure 2.3). This pattern occurs in respiratory failure caused by neuromus-

157

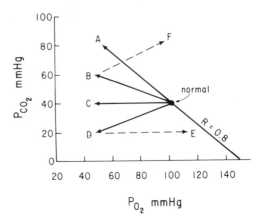

Figure 8.1. Patterns of arterial P_{O_2} and P_{CO_2} in different types of respiratory failure. Note that the P_{CO_2} can be high, as in pure hypoventilation (A), or low, as in the adult respiratory distress syndrome (D). The *broken lines* show the effects of oxygen breathing. (See text for further details.)

cular disease such as poliomyelitis, or an overdose of a narcotic drug (Figure 2.5). Severe ventilation-perfusion ratio inequality with alveolar ventilation inadequate to maintain a normal arterial P_{CO_2} results in movement along a line such as B. The hypoxemia is more severe in relation to the hypercapnia than in the case of pure hypoventilation. Such a pattern is frequently seen in the respiratory failure of chronic obstructive lung disease.

Severe interstitial disease sometimes results in movement along *line C*. Here there is increasingly severe hypoxemia but no CO_2 retention because of the raised ventilation. This pattern may be seen in advanced diffuse interstitial lung disease or sarcoidosis. Sometimes there is a rise in arterial P_{CO_2}, but this is typically less marked than in obstructive diseases.

In respiratory failure caused by the adult respiratory distress syndrome ("shock lung"), the arterial P_{CO_2} is typically low, as shown by *line D*, but the hypoxemia may be extreme. Such patients are usually treated with added inspired oxygen, which raises the arterial P_{O_2} but does not usually affect the P_{CO_2} (D to E). Oxygen therapy to patients whose respiratory failure is caused by chronic obstructive lung disease improves the arterial P_{O_2} but frequently causes a rise in P_{CO_2} because of depression of ventilation (B to F).

Hypoxemia of Respiratory Failure

Causes

Any of the four mechanisms of hypoxemia—hypoventilation, diffusion impairment, shunt, and ventilation-perfusion inequality—can contribute to the severe hypoxemia of respiratory failure. However, by far the most important cause is ventilation-perfusion inequality (including blood flow through unventilated lung). This is largely responsible for the low arterial P_{O_2} in respiratory failure complicating obstructive diseases, restrictive diseases, and the adult respiratory distress syndrome.

Detection

Severe hypoxemia causes cyanosis, cardiovascular signs such as tachycardia, and central nervous system effects such as mental clouding. However, a discussion of the detection of hypoxemia from these signs is largely academic because measurement of the P_{O_2} in the arterial blood is essential in determining the degree of hypoxemia in patients with suspected respiratory failure.

Tissue Hypoxia

Hypoxemia is dangerous because it causes tissue hypoxia. However, it is important to remember that the arterial P_{O_2} is only one factor in the delivery of oxygen to the tissues. Other factors include the oxygen capacity of the blood, the oxygen affinity of the hemoglobin, cardiac output, and the distribution of blood flow (pages 177–178).

Tissues vary considerably in their vulnerability to hypoxia. Those at greatest risk include the central nervous system and the myocardium. Cessation of blood flow to the cerebral cortex results in loss of function within 4–6 sec, loss of consciousness in 10–20 sec, and irreversible changes in 3–5 min.

If the P_{O_2} falls below a critical level in tissue, aerobic oxidation ceases and anaerobic glycolysis takes over with the formation and release of increasing amounts of lactic acid. The P_{O_2} at which this occurs is not accurately known and probably varies between tissues. However, there is some evidence that the critical intracellular P_{O_2} is of the order of 1 mm Hg in the region of the mitochondria.

Anaerobic glycolysis is a relatively inefficient method of obtaining energy from glucose. Nevertheless, it plays a critical role in maintaining tissue viability in respiratory failure. The large amounts of lactic acid which are formed are released into the blood, causing a metabolic acidosis. If tissue oxygenation subsequently improves, the lactic acid can be reconverted to glucose or used directly for energy. Most of this reconversion takes place in the liver.

Effects of Severe Hypoxemia

Mild hypoxemia produces few physiological changes. It should be recalled that the arterial oxygen saturation is still about 90% when the P_{O_2} is only 60 mm Hg (Figure 2.2) at a normal pH. The only abnormalities are a slight impairment of mental performance and visual acuity and mild hyperventilation.

When the arterial P_{O_2} drops quickly below 40–50 mm Hg, deleterious effects are seen in several organ systems. The central nervous system is particularly vulnerable and the patient often has headache, somnolence, or clouding of consciousness. Profound acute hypoxemia may cause convulsions, retinal hemorrhages, and permanent brain damage. The cardiovascular system shows tachycardia and mild hypertension, partly due to the release of catecholamines; in very severe hypoxemia there may be bradycardia and hypotension. Signs of heart failure may occur if there is associated coronary heart disease. Renal function is impaired and sodium retention and proteinuria may be seen. Pulmonary hypertension is common because of the associated alveolar hypoxia.

Hypercapnia in Respiratory Failure

Causes

Both of the two mechanisms of CO_2 retention—hypoventilation and ventilation-perfusion inequality—can be important in respiratory failure. Hypoventilation is the cause in respiratory failure due to neuromuscular diseases such as the Guillain-Barré syndrome, drug overdosage such as barbiturate poisoning, or a chest wall abnormality such as crushed chest (Figure 2.5). Ventilation-perfusion inequality is the culprit in severe chronic obstructive lung disease and long-standing interstitial disease.

An important cause of CO_2 retention in respiratory failure is the injudicious use of oxygen therapy. Many patients with chronic obstructive lung disease gradually develop severe hypoxemia and some CO_2 retention over a period of months. It is not customary to refer to this situation as respiratory failure because these patients can continue in this state for long periods. However, such a patient usually has a high work of breathing (Figures 3.3B and 4.12), and much of his ventilatory drive comes from hypoxic stimulation of the peripheral chemoreceptors. The arterial pH is virtually normal because of renal retention of bicarbonate (compensated respiratory acidosis), and the pH of the CSF is also normal because of an increase in bicarbonate there. Thus, in spite of an increased arterial P_{CO_2}, the main ventilatory drive comes from the hypoxemia.

If this patient develops a relatively mild intercurrent respiratory infection and is treated with a high inspired oxygen concentration, a potentially dangerous situation can rapidly develop. His hypoxic ventilatory drive may be abolished while his work of breathing is increased due to retained secretions or bronchospasm. As a result, the ventilation may become grossly depressed and very high levels of arterial P_{CO_2} may develop. In addition, profound hypoxemia may ensue if the oxygen is discontinued. This is because even if the ventilation does return to its previous level, the patient may take many minutes to unload the large accumulation of CO_2 in his tissues due to the large body stores of this gas.

A secondary cause of CO_2 retention in these patients may be the release of hypoxic vasoconstriction in poorly ventilated areas of lung as a result of the increased alveolar P_{O_2}. The consequences of this are increased blood flow to low $\dot{V}A/\dot{Q}$ areas and a worsening of $\dot{V}A/\dot{Q}$ inequality which exaggerates the CO_2 retention. This factor is probably less important than the depression of ventilation, but the very rapid rise in arterial P_{CO_2} which is seen when some of these patients are given oxygen suggests that this mechanism may play a part.

Such patients present a therapeutic dilemma. On the one hand oxygen administration is likely to cause severe CO_2 retention and respiratory acidosis. On the other hand it is clearly essential to give some oxygen to relieve the life-threatening hypoxemia. The answer to this problem is to give a relatively low concentration (24–28% O_2) and to monitor the arterial blood gases frequently to determine whether or not depression of ventilation is occurring. This subject is discussed further in Chapter 9.

Effects

Raised levels of P_{CO_2} in the blood greatly increase cerebral blood flow, causing headache, raised CSF pressure, and, sometimes, papilledema. In practice the cerebral effects of hypercapnia overlap with the effects of hypoxemia. The resulting abnormalities include restlessness, tremor, slurred speech, asterixis (flapping tremor), and fluctuations of mood. High levels of P_{CO_2} are narcotic and cause clouding of consciousness.

Acidosis in Respiratory Failure

The CO_2 retention causes a respiratory acidosis which may be very severe, especially following the injudicious administration of oxygen. However, patients who gradually develop respiratory failure may retain considerable amounts of bicarbonate, keeping the fall of pH in check (Figure 2.12).

Metabolic acidosis frequently coexists with respiratory acidosis and complicates the acid-base abnormality. This is caused by the liberation of lactic acid from hypoxic tissues, and the dual factors of hypoxemia and an inadequate peripheral circulation are additive. In patients who are mechanically ventilated, the raised intrathoracic pressure may interfere with venous return and cardiac output and thus further reduce peripheral blood flow (Figure 10.6).

Role of Diaphragm Fatigue

Recently, there has been increasing interest in the possible contribution of fatigue of the diaphragm to the hypoventilation of respiratory failure. The diaphragm consists of striated skeletal muscle controlled by voluntary and automatic neural pathways via the phrenic nerves. Although it is made up predominantly of slow twitch oxidative and fast twitch oxidative glycolytic fibers which are relatively resistant to fatigue, this can occur if the work of breathing is greatly increased over prolonged periods of time. Fatigue can be defined as a loss of contractile force after work, and can be measured from the transdiaphragmatic pressure resulting from a maximum contraction, or indirectly from the muscle relaxation time or the electromyogram. There is evidence that some patients with severe chronic obstructive lung disease continually breathe close to the work level at which fatigue occurs, and that an exacerbation of infection can tip them over into a fatigue state. This will then result in hypoventilation, CO_2 retention, and severe hypoxemia. Since hypercapnia impairs diaphragm contractility and severe hypoxemia accelerates the onset of fatigue, a vicious circle develops.

The dangers of diaphragm fatigue can be limited by reducing the work of breathing by treating bronchospasm and controlling infection, and by giving oxygen judiciously to relieve the hypoxemia. The force of contraction can be improved by a training program, for example, by breathing through inspiratory resistances. In addition, the administration of methylxanthines improves diaphragm contractility and since these drugs also relieve reversible bronchoconstriction, they are frequently employed. However, the role of fatigue of the diaphragm in respiratory failure is still not fully understood.

TYPES OF RESPIRATORY FAILURE

A large number of conditions can lead to respiratory failure, and various classifications are possible. However, from the point of view of the physiological principles of management, five groups can be distinguished:

1. Acute overwhelming lung disease
2. Neuromuscular disorders
3. Acute on chronic lung disease
4. Adult respiratory distress syndrome
5. Infant respiratory distress syndrome

Acute Overwhelming Lung Disease

Many acute diseases, if severe enough, can lead to respiratory failure. These include infections such as fulminating viral or bacterial pneumonias, vascular diseases such as pulmonary embolism, and exposure to inhaled toxic substances such as chlorine gas or oxides of nitrogen. Respiratory failure supervenes as the primary disease progresses and profound hypoxemia with or without hypercapnia develops. Oxygen administration is required for the hypoxemia and mechanical ventilation may be necessary to tide the patient over the worst stage. A few patients have been treated by extracorporeal membrane oxygenators which largely take over the gas exchange function of the lung, but the results are disappointing. Treatment of the underlying disease, for example, antibiotics for bacterial pneumonias, is clearly necessary.

Neuromuscular Disorders

Respiratory failure may occur when the respiratory center is depressed by drugs such as heroin and barbiturates. Other conditions include central nervous system and neuromuscular diseases such as encephalitis, poliomyelitis, Guillain-Barré syndrome, myasthenia gravis, anticholinesterase poisoning, and progressive muscular dystrophy (Figure 2.5). Trauma to the chest wall can also be responsible.

In these conditions the essential feature is hypoventilation leading to CO_2 retention with moderate hypoxemia (Figures 2.3, 2.4, and 8.1). Respiratory acidosis occurs, but the magnitude of the fall in pH depends on the rapidity of the increase in P_{CO_2} and the extent of the renal compensation.

Mechanical ventilation is often necessary in these conditions and occasionally, as in bulbar poliomyelitis, it may be required for months or even years. However, the lung itself is often normal and, if so, no additional oxygen is necessary to reverse the hypoxemia. Again, treatment of the underlying disease is always indicated, if available.

Acute on Chronic Lung Disease

This is an important and common group which includes patients with chronic bronchitis and emphysema, asthma and cystic fibrosis. Many patients with chronic obstructive lung disease follow a gradual downhill course with increasingly severe hypoxemia and CO_2 retention over months or years. Such patients are usually capable of limited physical activity even though both the arterial P_{O_2} and P_{CO_2} may be in the region of 50 mm Hg. As a result this situation is not conventionally referred to as respiratory failure.

However, if such a patient develops even a mild exacerbation of his chest infection, his condition often deteriorates rapidly, with profound hypoxemia, CO_2 retention, and respiratory acidosis. The reason is that his reserves of pulmonary function are minimal, and any increase in the work of breathing or worsening of ventilation-perfusion relationships as a result of retained secretions or bronchospasm pushes him over the brink into frank respiratory failure.

The management of these patients requires a delicate touch. Naturally the underlying infection should be treated with antibiotics. In addition, bronchodilators may be indicated for bronchospasm, and diuretics and digitalis may be required if there is evidence of heart failure. Supplemental oxygen is necessary to relieve the severe hypoxemia. However, these patients frequently lose their ventilatory drive and develop very severe CO_2 retention and acidosis if too much oxygen is administered. For this reason it is usual to begin with 24–28% oxygen and monitor the arterial blood gases frequently (see page 161 and Chapter 9).

Mechanical ventilation may be necessary, but the decision to employ this is often a difficult one. On the one hand, it may be impossible to prevent the rise of arterial P_{CO_2} without artificial ventilation. On the other hand, these patients often have such diseased lungs that once they are on the ventilator, it may be impossible to wean them from it. Each case must be considered on its own merits, but mechanical ventilation should generally only be used if there is a substantial reversible component to the patient's condition.

Adult Respiratory Distress Syndrome

This condition is also known as "acute respiratory failure." The older terms "shock lung" and "post-traumatic wet lung" are now infrequently used. It is an end result of a variety of insults including trauma to the lung or to the rest of the body, septicemia, especially that caused by gram-negative organisms, and shock from any cause (40).

Pathology

The early changes consist of interstitial and alveolar edema. Hemorrhage, cellular debris, and proteinaceous fluid are present in the alveoli, hyaline membranes may be seen, and there is patchy atelectasis (Figure 8.2) (41). Later, hyperplasia and organization occur. The damaged alveolar epithelium becomes lined with type 2 alveolar cells and there is cellular infiltration of the alveolar walls. Eventually interstitial fibrosis may develop, although complete healing can occur.

The cause of the changes is unknown but there is evidence that the permeability of the blood-gas barrier is increased. For example, the alveolar fluid contains large amounts of protein, and leakage into the alveoli of intravenously administered dextran of high molecular weight (up to 500,000) has been demonstrated in some patients (33).

Clinical Features

A feature of the condition is that it is often associated with some severe underlying medical or surgical illness unconnected with the

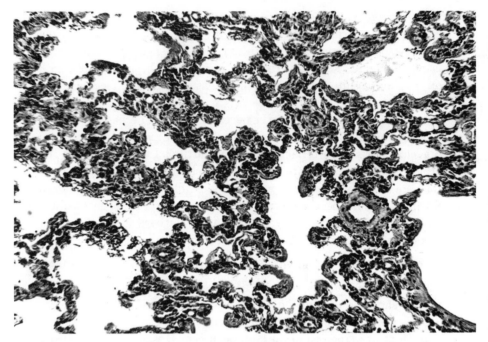

Figure 8.2. Histological changes in the adult respiratory distress syndrome as found by an open lung biopsy. Note the patchy atelectasis, edema, and cellular debris in the alveoli. (From M. Lamy, R. J. Fallat, E. Koeniger, H.-P. Dietrich, J. L. Ratliff, R. C. Eberhart, H. J. Tucker, and J. D. Hill: Pathologic features and mechanisms of hypoxemia in adult respiratory distress syndrome. *Am. Rev. Respir. Dis.* 114:267–284, 1976 (41).)

lung and the onset of respiratory failure is often delayed. A typical history is that the patient is exposed to severe trauma, for example, an automobile accident with multiple fractures. There is some hemorrhagic shock with hypotension which is treated by fluid replacement. He appears to be doing well when, perhaps 2 days after the trauma, some increase in respiratory rate is noted, the arterial P_{O_2} and P_{CO_2} fall, and clouding is seen in the chest radiograph. Severe hypoxemia then develops. The mortality is around 50%.

Pulmonary Function

The lung becomes very stiff and unusually high pressures are required to ventilate the lung with a respirator. Associated with this reduced compliance is a marked fall in FRC. The cause of the increased recoil is presumably the alveolar edema and exudate, which exaggerate the surface tension forces. As was pointed out earlier (Figure 6.3), edematous alveoli have a reduced volume. It is also possible that interstitial edema contributes to the abnormal stiffness of the lungs.

As would be expected from the histological appearance of the lung (Figure 8.2), there is marked ventilation-perfusion inequality, with a substantial fraction of the total blood flow going to unventilated alveoli. This fraction may reach 50% or more. Figure 8.3 shows some results obtained by the multiple inert gas method in a 44-year-old patient who developed respiratory failure after an automobile accident and was mechanically ventilated. Note the presence of blood flow to lung units with abnormally low ventilation-perfusion ratios and also the shunt of 8% (compare the normal distribution in Figure 2.10). Figure 8.3 also shows a large amount of ventilation going to units with high ventilation-perfusion ratios. One reason for this is the abnormally high airway pressures developed by the ventilator, which reduces the blood flow in some alveoli (compare Figure 10.4).

The ventilation-perfusion inequality and shunt cause profound hy-

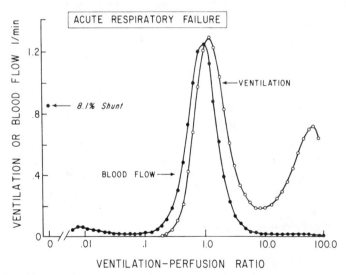

Figure 8.3. Distribution of ventilation-perfusion ratios in a patient who developed the adult respiratory distress syndrome following an automobile accident. Note the 8% shunt and the blood flow to units with low ventilation-perfusion ratios. In addition, there is some ventilation to high $\dot{V}A/\dot{Q}$ units, probably as a result of the high airway pressure developed by the ventilator (compare Figure 10.4).

poxemia. Usually these patients must be given enriched oxygen mixtures because air breathing even with a respirator results in an arterial P_{O_2} which is dangerously low. Oxygen concentrations of 40–100% are sometimes necessary during mechanical ventilation to maintain an arterial P_{O_2} above 60 mm Hg. The addition of positive end-expiratory pressure (PEEP) often results in a substantial improvement in oxygenation in these patients (compare Figure 10.4).

By contrast, the arterial P_{CO_2} is typically low even when severe hypoxemia develops, values in the 20's being common. The reason for the increased ventilation is not known, though possibly the interstitial edema stimulates intrapulmonary J or stretch receptors. Another possible factor is stimulation of the peripheral chemoreceptors by the hypoxemia, though relieving this does not usually affect the level of ventilation.

Infant Respiratory Distress Syndrome

This condition, which is also called hyaline membrane disease of the newborn, has several features in common with the adult respiratory distress syndrome just discussed (42). Pathologically, the lung shows hemorrhagic edema, patchy atelectasis, and hyaline membranes caused by proteinaceous fluid and cellular debris within the alveoli. Physiologically there is profound hypoxemia, with both ventilation-perfusion inequality and blood flow through unventilated lung. In addition a right-to-left shunt via the patent foramen ovale may exaggerate the hypoxemia. Mechanical ventilation with enriched oxygen mixtures is often necessary and the addition of PEEP or continuous positive airway pressure (see Chapter 10) is frequently beneficial.

The chief cause of this condition is an absence of pulmonary surfactant, though other factors are also probably involved. The surfactant is normally produced by the type 2 alveolar cells (Figure 5.2), and the ability of the lung to synthesize adequate amounts of the material develops relatively late in fetal life. Thus, a prematurely born infant is particularly at risk. The ability of the infant to secrete surfactant can be estimated by measuring the lecithin/sphingomyelin ratio of amniotic fluid, and there is some evidence that maturation of the surfactant-synthesizing system can be hastened by the administration of corticosteroids. Treatment of the condition by administering animal or human surfactant to the lung appears promising.

MANAGEMENT OF RESPIRATORY FAILURE

Although many factors enter into the management of an individual patient, it is useful to discuss the physiological principles underlying treatment. Naturally, attention must be directed to the primary cause of the disease. For example, antibiotic therapy may be required for an infection, or a specific treatment may be available for a neuromuscular disorder. However, some aspects of management are common to many patients with respiratory failure.

Airway Obstruction

Respiratory failure is often precipitated by an increase in airway resistance. Many patients have chronic obstructive lung disease of many years' duration with hypoxemia and even some mild hypercapnia. Even so they are able to maintain a little physical activity. However, if they develop bronchospasm through exposure to smog or cold air or they have a "chesty cold" with an increase in secretions, they may rapidly develop respiratory faiure. The additional work of breathing becomes the straw that breaks the camel's back and they develop profound hypoxemia, CO_2 retention, and respiratory acidosis.

Treatment should be directed at reducing the airway obstruction. Retained secretions are best removed by coughing when this is effective. Encouragement to cough and assistance by a respiratory therapist, nurse, or physician is often helpful, and changing the patient's position from side to side to assist drainage of secretions may be beneficial. Adequate hydration is important to prevent the secretions from becoming too viscid. It is especially important to humidify all gases given by a ventilator to prevent thickening and crusting of secretions. Drugs such as potassium iodide by mouth or acetylcysteine by aerosol to liquefy sputum are of doubtful value. Aspiration of secretions by bronchoscopy may become necessary. Occasionally, respiratory stimulants are given to a drowsy patient but, more importantly, respiratory depressants must be avoided because they suppress coughing.

Any reversible airway obstruction should be treated by bronchodilators such as salbutamol or metaproterenol aerosol, intravenous aminophylline, or perhaps, intravenous corticosteroids. Drugs such as isoproterenol, which stimulate β_1-adrenergic receptors in the heart, are less valuable than drugs which mainly stimulate β_2-receptors in the lung because of the dangers of inducing abnormal rhythms in a hypoxic myocardium.

Respiratory Infection

An exacerbation of existing bronchitis in a patient with chronic obstructive lung disease, or a fresh respiratory infection in a patient with advanced interstitial lung disease, frequently provokes respiratory failure. There are at least two physiological mechanisms for this. First, the increased secretions and, perhaps, bronchospasm increase the work of breathing as discussed above. Second, there is a worsening of ventilation-perfusion relationships, so that even if the ventilation to the alveoli remains unchanged, there will be increasing hypoxemia and hypercapnia. Treatment of the infection by antibiotics is indicated.

It should be pointed out that even a mild exacerbation of bronchitis in a patient with chronic obstructive lung disease may precipitate respiratory failure. Moreover, the usual systemic responses to infection such as pyrexia and leukocytosis are often absent. However, treatment should not be delayed.

Cardiac Insufficiency

Many patients with incipient respiratory failure have a compromised cardiovascular system. The pulmonary artery pressure is frequently raised, as a result of several factors, including destruction of the pulmonary capillary bed by disease, hypoxic vasoconstriction, and increased blood viscosity caused by polycythemia. In addition, the myocardium is chronically hypoxic. Fluid retention often occurs as a result of retention of bicarbonate and sodium ions by the hypoxic kidney. Finally, some patients have coexisting coronary artery disease.

Patients with chronic obstructive lung disease frequently develop peripheral edema, hepatomegaly, and engorged neck veins. These and other patients may also show signs of left heart failure, with basal rales (crackles) on auscultation and engorged lung fields on the radiograph. The mild pulmonary edema will further interfere with pulmonary gas exchange by causing uneven ventilation. Treatment with diuretics and digitalis is then indicated.

Hypoxemia

This can be relieved to some extent by treating the airway obstruction and the chest infection. However, the administration of long-term oxygen is frequently required, and this important topic is discussed in detail in Chapter 9.

Hypercapnia

Again this often responds to general measures directed at the airway obstruction and the infection. However, frequently mechanical ventilation is required. This is discussed in detail in Chapter 10.

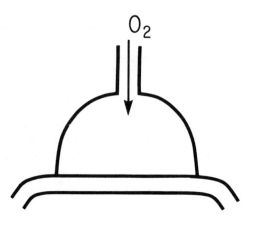

chapter 9

Oxygen Therapy

Oxygen administration has a critical role in the treatment of hypoxemia and, especially, in the management of respiratory failure. However, patients vary considerably in their response to oxygen, and there are several potential hazards associated with its use. A clear understanding of the physiological principles involved is necessary to prevent abuses of this powerful agent.

IMPROVED OXYGENATION FOLLOWING OXYGEN ADMINISTRATION

Power of Added Oxygen

The great extent to which the arterial P_{O_2} can be increased by the inhalation of 100% of oxygen is sometimes not appreciated. Suppose a young man has taken an overdose of a narcotic drug resulting in severe hypoventilation with an arterial P_{O_2} of 50 and a P_{CO_2} of 80 mm Hg (Figure 2.3). If this patient is mechanically ventilated and given 100% oxygen, the arterial P_{O_2} may increase to over 600 mm Hg; that is a 10-fold increase (Figure 9.1). There are not many drugs that can change the gas exchange of the blood so much so effortlessly!

172

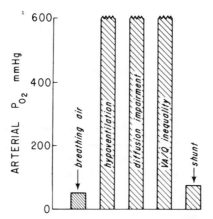

Figure 9.1. Response of the arterial P_{O_2} to 100% inspired oxygen for the different mechanisms of hypoxemia. The P_{O_2} breathing air is assumed to be 50 mm Hg. Note the dramatic increase in all instances except shunt where, nevertheless, there is a useful gain.

Response of Various Types of Hypoxemia

The mechanism of hypoxemia has an important bearing on its response to inhaled oxygen.

Hypoventilation

The rise in alveolar P_{O_2} can be predicted from the alveolar gas equation *if* the ventilation and metabolic rate, and therefore the alveolar P_{CO_2}, remain unaltered:

$$PA_{O_2} = PI_{O_2} - \frac{PA_{CO_2}}{R} + F$$

where F is a small correction factor.

Assuming no change in the alveolar P_{CO_2} and the respiratory exchange ratio and neglecting the correction factor, this equation shows that the alveolar P_{O_2} rises parallel with the inspired value. Thus, changing from air to only 30% oxygen can increase the alveolar P_{O_2} by about 60 mm Hg. In practice the arterial P_{O_2} will always be lower than the alveolar value because of a small amount of venous admixture. However, it is clear that the hypoxemia of hypoventilation, which is rarely severe (Figures 2.3 and 2.14), is very easily reversed by a modest oxygen enrichment of the inspired gas.

Diffusion Impairment

Again, hypoxemia due to this mechanism is readily overcome by oxygen administration. The reason for this becomes clear if we look at the dynamics of oxygen uptake along the pulmonary capillary (Figure 2.6). The rate of movement of oxygen across the blood-gas barrier is proportional to the P_{O_2} difference between alveolar gas and capillary blood.* This difference is normally about 60 mm Hg at the beginning of the capillary. Now if we increase the concentration of inspired oxygen to only 30%, we raise the alveolar P_{O_2} by 60 mm Hg, thus doubling the rate of transfer of oxygen at the start of the capillary. This in turn improves oxygenation of the end-capillary blood. Thus again, a very modest rise in inspired oxygen concentration can usually correct the hypoxemia.

Ventilation-Perfusion Inequality

Again, oxygen administration is usually very effective at improving the arterial P_{O_2}. However, the rise in P_{O_2} depends on the pattern of ventilation-perfusion inequality and the inspired oxygen concentration. Administration of 100% O_2 increases the arterial P_{O_2} to very high values because every lung unit which is ventilated eventually washes out its nitrogen. When this occurs, the alveolar P_{O_2} is given by: $P_{O_2} = P_B - P_{H_2O} - P_{CO_2}$. Since the P_{CO_2} is normally less than 50 mm Hg, this equation predicts an alveolar P_{O_2} of over 600 mm Hg, even in lung units with very low ventilation-perfusion ratios, as is shown in Figure 9.2.

However, two cautions should be added. First, some regions of the lung may be so poorly ventilated that it may take many minutes for the nitrogen to be washed out. Furthermore, these regions may continue to receive nitrogen, as this gas is gradually washed out of peripheral tissues by the venous blood. As a consequence, the arterial P_{O_2} may take so long to reach its final level that in practice this is never achieved. Second, giving oxygen may result in the development of unventilated areas (Figure 9.6). If this occurs, the rise in arterial P_{O_2} will stop short (Figure 9.4).

When intermediate concentrations of oxygen are given, the rise in

---

* See J. B. West: *Respiratory Physiology—The Essentials*, ed. 3, p. 24. Baltimore, Williams & Wilkins, 1985.

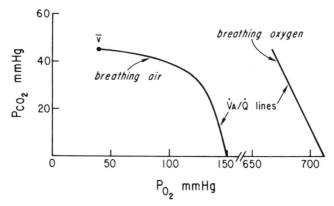

Figure 9.2. O_2-CO_2 diagram showing typical ventilation-perfusion ratio lines during the breathing of air and 100% oxygen. Note that in the latter case the alveolar P_{O_2} remains extremely high for all values of ventilation-perfusion ratios. (The mixed venous point $\bar{v}$ refers to air breathing only.)

arterial P_{O_2} is determined by the pattern of ventilation-perfusion inequality and in particular by those units which have very low ventilation-perfusion ratios and appreciable blood flow. Figure 9.3 shows the response of the arterial P_{O_2} in lung models with various distributions of ventilation-perfusion ratios after inspiration of various oxygen concentrations (43). Note that at an inspired concentration of 60%, the arterial P_{O_2} of the distribution with a standard deviation of 2.0 rose from 40 to only 90 mm Hg. This modest rise can be attributed to the effects of lung units with ventilation-perfusion ratios less than 0.01. For example, an alveolus with a ventilation-perfusion ratio of 0.006 which is given 60% O_2 to inspire has an end-capillary P_{O_2} of only 60 mm Hg in the example shown. However, note that when the inspired oxygen concentration was increased to 90%, the arterial P_{O_2} of this distribution rose to nearly 500 mm Hg.

Figure 9.3 assumes that the pattern of ventilation-perfusion inequality remains constant as the inspired oxygen is raised. However, the relief of alveolar hypoxia in poorly ventilated regions of lung may increase the blood flow there because of the abolition of hypoxic vasoconstriction. In this case the increase in arterial P_{O_2} will be less. Note also that if units with low ventilation-perfusion ratios collapse during high oxygen breathing (Figures 9.6 and 9.7), the arterial P_{O_2} will rise less.

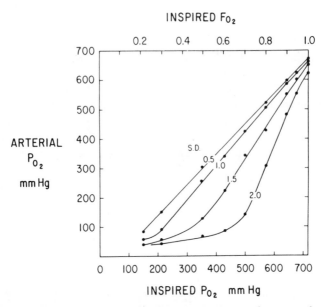

Figure 9.3. Response of the arterial P_{O_2} to various inspired oxygen values in theoretical distributions of ventilation-perfusion ratios. SD refers to the standard deviation of the log normal distribution. Note that when the distribution is very broad (SD = 2), the arterial P_{O_2} remains low even when 60% oxygen is inhaled. (From J. B. West and P. D. Wagner: Pulmonary gas exchange. In J. B. West (ed.): *Bioengineering Aspects of the Lung.* New York, Marcel Dekker, 1977 (43).)

Shunt

This is the only mechanism of hypoxemia where the arterial P_{O_2} remains way below the level for the normal lung during 100% O_2 breathing. The reason is that the blood which bypasses the ventilated alveoli (shunt) does not "see" the added oxygen and, being low in oxygen content, depresses the arterial P_{O_2}. This depression is particularly marked because of the very shallow slope of the oxygen dissociation curve at a high P_{O_2} (Figure 2.8).

However, it should be emphasized that useful gains in arterial P_{O_2} often follow the administration of 100% O_2 to patients with shunts. This is because of the additional dissolved oxygen, which can be appreciable at a high alveolar P_{O_2}. For example, increasing the alveolar P_{O_2} from 100 to 600 mm Hg raises the dissolved oxygen in the end capillary blood from 0.3 to 1.8 ml of O_2/100 ml of blood. This increase of 1.5 can be compared with the normal arterial-venous difference in oxygen content of about 5 ml/100 ml.

Figure 9.4 shows typical increases in arterial P_{O_2} for various percentage shunts at different inspired oxygen concentrations. The graph is drawn for an oxygen uptake of 300 ml/min and cardiac output of 6 liters/min; variations in these and other values will alter the positions of the lines. However, note that in this example, a patient with a 30% shunt who has an arterial P_{O_2} of 55 mm Hg during air breathing will increase this to 110 mm Hg if he breathes 100% oxygen. This corresponds to a rise in oxygen saturation and content of the arterial blood of 10% and 2.2 ml/100 ml, respectively. In a patient with a hypoxic myocardium, for example, these values mean an important gain in oxygen delivery.

Other Factors in Oxygen Delivery

Although the arterial P_{O_2} is a very convenient measurement of the degree of oxygenation of the blood, it should be emphasized again that other factors are important in oxygen delivery to the tissues (see also page 34). The factors include the hemoglobin concentration, the po-

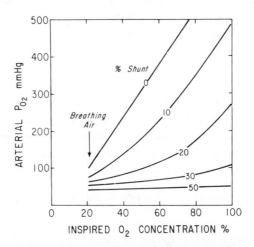

Figure 9.4. Response of the arterial P_{O_2} to increased inspired oxygen concentrations in a lung with various amounts of shunt. Note that the P_{O_2} remains a long way below the normal level for 100% oxygen. Nevertheless, useful gains in oxygenation occur even with severe degrees of shunting. (This diagram shows typical values only; changes in cardiac output, oxygen uptake, etc., will affect the position of the lines.)

sition of the oxygen dissociation curve, the cardiac output, and its distribution throughout the peripheral tissues.

Both a fall in hemoglobin concentration and cardiac output reduce the total amount of oxygen per unit time ("oxygen flux") going to the tissues. The flux may be expressed as the product of the cardiac output and the arterial oxygen content: $\dot{Q} \cdot Ca_{O_2}$.

Diffusion of oxygen from the peripheral capillaries to the mitochondria in the tissue cells depends on capillary P_{O_2}. A useful index is the P_{O_2} of mixed venous blood, which is close to the average tissue P_{O_2}. A rearrangement of the Fick equation

$$C_{\bar{v}_{O_2}} = C_{a_{O_2}} - \frac{\dot{V}_{O_2}}{\dot{Q}}$$

shows that the oxygen content (and therefore the P_{O_2}) of mixed venous blood will fall if either the arterial oxygen content or the cardiac output is reduced (oxygen consumption assumed constant).

The relationship between oxygen content and P_{O_2} in the mixed venous blood depends on the position of the oxygen dissociation curve (Figure 2.2). If the curve is shifted to the right by an increase in temperature, as in fever, or an increase in 2,3-DPG concentration as frequently occurs in chronic hypoxemia, the P_{O_2} for a given content will be high, thus favoring diffusion of oxygen to the mitochondria. By contrast, if the P_{CO_2} is low and the pH is high, as in respiratory alkalosis, or if the 2,3-DPG concentration is low because of transfusion of large amounts of stored blood, the resulting left-shifted curve interferes with oxygen unloading to the tissues.

Finally, the distribution of cardiac output clearly plays an important role in tissue oxygenation. For example, a patient with coronary artery disease is liable to have hypoxic regions in his myocardium, irrespective of the other factors involved in oxygen delivery.

METHODS OF OXYGEN ADMINISTRATION

Nasal Cannulas

These consist of two prongs which are inserted just inside the anterior nares and supported on a light frame. Oxygen is supplied at rates of 1–4 liters/min, resulting in inspired oxygen concentrations of about 25–30%. The higher the patient's inspiratory flow rate, the lower the resulting concentration. The gas should be humidified as close to body temperature as possible to prevent crusting of secretions on the nasal mucosa.

The chief advantage of cannulas is that the patient does not have the discomfort of a mask and he can talk and eat and has access to his face. The cannulas can be worn continuously for long periods, an important point because oxygen administration should usually be continuous rather than intermittent (see below). The disadvantages of cannulas are the low maximum inspired concentrations of oxygen which are available and the unpredictability of the concentration, especially if the patient breathes partly through his mouth.

Masks

There are several designs. Simple plastic masks which fit over the nose and mouth allow inspired oxygen concentrations of up to 60% when supplied with flow rates of 6 liters/min. However, because some accumulation of CO_2 occurs within the mask (up to 2%), this device is not suitable for patients who are liable to develop CO_2 retention. In addition, some patients complain of feeling smothered when this type of mask is used.

A useful mask for delivering controlled oxygen concentrations is based on the Venturi principle. As the oxygen enters the mask through a narrow jet, it entrains a constant flow of air, which enters via surrounding holes. With an oxygen flow of 4 liters/min, a total flow of (oxygen + air) of about 40 liters/min is delivered to the patient. At such high flow rates there is negligible rebreathing of expired gas and therefore no CO_2 accumulation. Masks which give inspired oxygen concentrations of 24, 28, or 35% with a high degree of reliability are available and are particularly useful for treating patients who are liable to develop CO_2 retention. Some patients complain of the noise and the breeze, while others enjoy the latter.

Tents

These are now only used for children who do not tolerate masks well. Oxygen concentrations of up to 50% can be obtained.

Ventilators

When a patient is mechanically ventilated through an endotracheal or tracheostomy tube, complete control over the composition of the inspired gas is available. There is a danger of producing oxygen toxicity if concentrations of over 50% are given for more than 2 days (see below). In general, the lowest inspired oxygen which provides an acceptable arterial P_{O_2} should be used. This is difficult to define, but in patients with the adult respiratory distress syndrome who are being mechanically ventilated with high oxygen concentrations, a figure of 60 mm Hg is often used.

Hyperbaric Oxygen

If 100% O_2 is administered at a pressure of 3 atmospheres, the inspired P_{O_2} is over 2000 mm Hg. Under these conditions a substantial increase in the arterial oxygen content can occur, chiefly as a result of additional dissolved oxygen. For example, if the arterial P_{O_2} is 2000 mm Hg, the oxygen in solution is about 6 ml/100 ml of blood. Theoretically this is enough to provide the entire arterial-venous difference of 5 ml/100 ml, so that the hemoglobin of the mixed venous blood could remain fully saturated.

Hyperbaric oxygen therapy has limited uses and is rarely indicated in the management of respiratory failure. However, it has been used in the treatment of severe carbon monoxide poisoning where most of the hemoglobin is unavailable to carry oxygen and therefore the dissolved oxygen is critically important. In addition, the high P_{O_2} accelerates the dissociation of carbon monoxide from hemoglobin. A severe anemic crisis is sometimes treated in the same way. Hyperbaric oxygen is also used in the treatment of gas gangrene infections and as an adjunct to radiotherapy where the higher tissue P_{O_2} increases the radiosensitivity of relatively avascular tumors. The high pressure chamber is also valuable for managing decompression sickness.

The use of hyperbaric oxygen requires a special facility with trained personnel. In practice the chamber is filled with air and oxygen is given by a special mask to ensure that the patient receives pure oxygen. This procedure also reduces fire hazard.

Domiciliary and Portable Oxygen

Some patients are so disabled by severe chronic lung disease that they are virtually confined to bed or a chair unless they breathe supplementary oxygen. These patients often benefit considerably from having a supply of oxygen in their home. This can take various forms. A central large tank with a long plastic tube and mask may enable the patient to climb stairs or go to the bathroom. In addition, portable oxygen sets are available, and these can even be used for shopping or other activities. Some sets use liquid oxygen as a store, while in others, oxygen is extracted from the air with a molecular sieve.

The patients who benefit most from portable oxygen are those whose exercise tolerance is limited by dyspnea. Increasing the inspired oxygen concentration can greatly increase the level of exercise for a given ventilation and so enable these patients to become much more active.

It has been shown that a low flow of oxygen given continuously over several months can reduce the amount of pulmonary hypertension and improve the prognosis of some patients with advanced chronic obstructive lung disease. Although such therapy is expensive, improvements in the technology of providing oxygen are making it increasingly feasible.

HAZARDS OF OXYGEN THERAPY

Carbon Dioxide Retention

The reasons for the development of dangerous CO_2 retention following oxygen administration to patients with severe chronic obstructive lung disease were briefly discussed in page 160. A critical factor in the ventilatory drive of these patients who have a high work of breathing is often the hypoxic stimulation of their peripheral chemoreceptors. If this is removed by relieving their hypoxemia, the level of ventilation may fall precipitously and severe CO_2 retention may ensue.

Intermittent oxygen therapy is especially dangerous. The physiologist Haldane compared this with bringing a drowning man to the surface—occasionally!

The explanation is that if oxygen administration is seen to cause CO_2 retention and is therefore stopped, the subsequent hypoxemia may be more severe than it was prior to oxygen therapy. The reason is the increased alveolar P_{CO_2} as can be seen from the alveolar gas equation:

$$P_{A_{O_2}} = P_{I_{O_2}} - \frac{P_{A_{CO_2}}}{R} + F$$

Moreover, the high P_{CO_2} is likely to remain for many minutes because the body stores of this gas are so great that the excess is only gradually washed out. Thus, the hypoxemia may be severe and prolonged.

These patients should be given continuous oxygen at a low concentration and the blood gases must be monitored. Initially an oxygen concentration of 24% is often given by means of a Venturi mask and the arterial P_{O_2} and P_{CO_2} are measured after 15–20 min. If the P_{CO_2} does not rise more than a few mm Hg and the patient remains alert, the oxygen concentration can be increased to 28%. This is generally adequate to relieve severe hypoxemia, though concentrations as high as 35% are sometimes used. The shape of the oxygen dissociation curve (Figure 2.2) should be at the back of the physician's mind to remind him that a rise in P_{O_2} from 30 to 50 mm Hg (at a normal pH) represents more than a 25% increase in hemoglobin saturation!

Oxygen Toxicity

High concentrations of oxygen over long periods damage the lung. Figure 9.5 shows an electron micrograph from a monkey exposed to 100% oxygen for 2 days (compare Figure 5.1) (44). Note the swollen capillary endothelium, which is where some of the earliest changes are seen. Alterations also occur in the endothelial intercellular junctions, resulting in an increased capillary permeability which leads to interstitial and alveolar edema. In addition, the alveolar epithelium may become completely denuded and replaced by rows of type 2 epithelial cells. Later, organization occurs, with interstitial fibrosis.

In man the pulmonary effects of high oxygen concentration are more difficult to document, but normal subjects complain of substernal discomfort after breathing 100% oxygen for 24 hr. Patients who have been mechanically ventilated with 100% oxygen for 36 hr have shown a progressive fall in arterial P_{O_2} compared with a control group who were ventilated with air. A reasonable attitude is to assume that concentrations of 50% or higher for more than 2 days may produce toxic changes.

Figure 9.5. Early changes in oxygen toxicity. This electron micrograph from a monkey exposed to 100% oxygen for 2 days shows swelling of the capillary endothelial cells. Later changes include loss of alveolar epithelium and subsequent interstitial fibrosis. *A*, alveolus; *EN*, endothelium; *EP*, epithelium; *IN*, interstitium; *RBC*, red blood cell. (From U. Kapanci, E. R. Weibel, H. P. Kaplan, and F. R. Robinson: Pathogenesis and reversibility of the pulmonary lesions of oxygen toxicity in monkeys. *Lab. Invest.* 20:101–118, 1969 (44).)

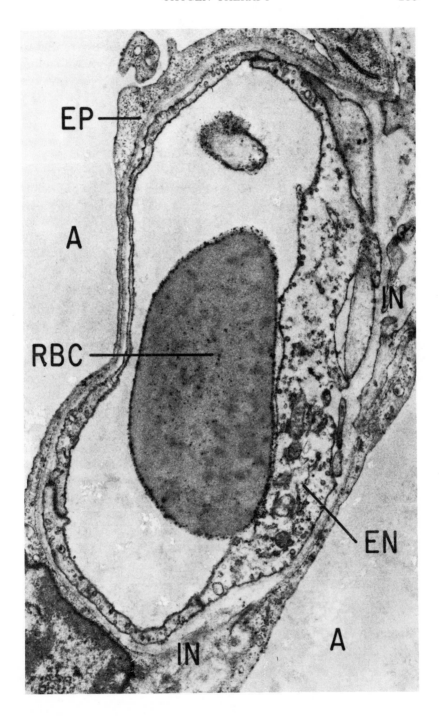

In practice such high levels over such a long period can only be achieved in patients who are intubated and mechanically ventilated. It is important to avoid oxygen toxicity because the only way to relieve the resultant hypoxemia is by raising the inspired oxygen, thus creating a vicious circle.

Atelectasis

Following Airway Occlusion

If a patient is breathing air and an airway becomes totally obstructed, for example, by retained secretions, absorption atelectasis of the lung behind the airway may occur. The reason is that the sum of the partial pressures in venous blood is considerably less than atmospheric pressure, with the result that the trapped gas is gradually absorbed.* However, the process is relatively slow, requiring many hours or even days.

On the other hand, if the patient is breathing a high concentration of oxygen, a rate of absorption atelectasis is greatly accelerated. This is because there is then relatively little nitrogen in the alveoli and this gas normally slows the absorption process because of its low solubility. Replacing the nitrogen with any other gas which is rapidly absorbed also predisposes to collapse. An example is nitrous oxide during anesthesia. In the normal lung, collateral ventilation may delay or prevent atelectasis by providing an alternate path for gas to enter the obstructed region (Figure 1.11C).

Absorption atelectasis is common in patients with respiratory failure because they often have excessive secretions or cellular debris in their airways and they are frequently treated with high oxygen concentrations. In addition the channels through which collateral ventilation normally occurs may be obstructed by disease. Collapse is common in the dependent regions of the lung because secretions tend to collect there, and those airways and alveoli are relatively poorly expanded anyway (Figure 3.5). To the extent that atelectatic lung is perfused, hypoxemia develops, though hypoxic vasoconstriction may limit this.

Instability of Units with Low Ventilation-Perfusion Ratios

It has been shown that lung units with low ventilation-perfusion ratios may become unstable and collapse when high oxygen mixtures are

* See J. B. West: *Respiratory Physiology—The Essentials*, ed. 3, p. 134. Baltimore, Williams & Wilkins, 1985.

inhaled. An example is given in Figure 9.6, which shows the distribution of ventilation-perfusion ratios in a patient during air breathing and after 30 min of 100% oxygen. This patient had respiratory failure following an automobile accident (Figure 8.3). Note that during air breathing there were appreciable amounts of blood flow to lung units with low ventilation-perfusion ratios in addition to an 8% shunt. After oxygen administration, the blood flow to the low ventilation-perfusion ratio units was not evident, but the shunt had increased to 16%. The most likely explanation of this change is that the poorly ventilated regions became unventilated.

Figure 9.7 shows the mechanism involved. The figure shows four hypothetical lung units, all with very low inspired ventilation-perfusion ratios ($\dot{V}_{AI}/\dot{Q}$) during 80% oxygen breathing. In A the inspired (alveolar) ventilation is 49.4 units but the expired ventilation is only 2.5 units (the actual values depend on the blood flow). The reason why so little gas is exhaled is that so much is taken up by the blood. In B, where the inspired ventilation is slightly reduced to 44.0 units

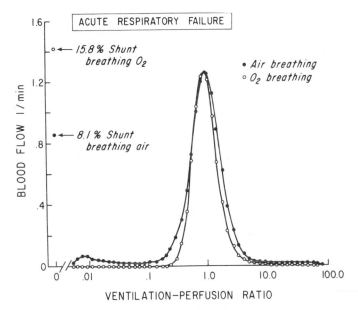

Figure 9.6. Conversion of low ventilation-perfusion ratio units to shunt during oxygen breathing. This patient had respiratory failure following an automobile accident (same patient as shown in Figure 8.3). During air breathing there was appreciable blood flow to units with low ventilation-perfusion ratios. Following 30 min of 100% oxygen, these units were not evident, but the shunt doubled.

INSPIRED O_2 = 80%

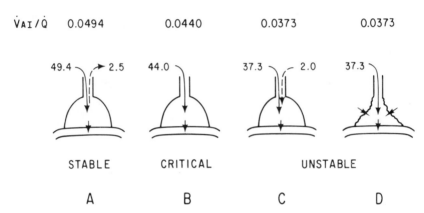

Figure 9.7. Mechanism of the collapse of lung units with low inspired ventilation-perfusion ratios ($\dot{V}_{AI}/\dot{Q}$) when high oxygen mixtures are inhaled. (*A*) The expired ventilation is very small because so much of the inspired gas is taken up by the blood. (*C* and *D*) More gas is removed from the lung unit than is inspired, leading to an unstable condition.

(same blood flow as before), there is no expired ventilation because all the gas which is inspired is absorbed by the blood. Such a unit is said to have a "critical" ventilation-perfusion ratio.

In *C* and *D*, the inspired ventilation has been further reduced with the result that it is now less than the volume of gas entering the blood. This is an unstable situation. Under these circumstances, either gas is inspired from neighboring units during the expiratory phase of respiration as in *C*, or the unit will gradually collapse as in *D*. The latter fate is particularly likely if the unit is poorly ventilated because of intermittent airway closure. This is probably common in the dependent regions of the lung in the adult respiratory distress syndrome because of the greatly reduced FRC. The likelihood of atelectasis increases rapidly as the inspired oxygen concentration approaches 100%.

The development of shunts during oxygen breathing is an additional reason why high concentrations of this gas should be avoided if possible in the treatment of patients with respiratory failure. Also, it should be recognized that the shunt which is measured during 100% oxygen breathing (Figure 2.8) in these patients may substantially overestimate the shunt which is present during air breathing.

Retrolental Fibroplasia

If newborn infants with the infant respiratory distress syndrome are treated with high concentrations of oxygen, they may develop fibrosis behind the lens of the eye, leading to blindness. This has been successfully avoided by keeping the arterial P_{O_2} below 140 mm Hg. However, recently the disease has reappeared for reasons that are not clear.

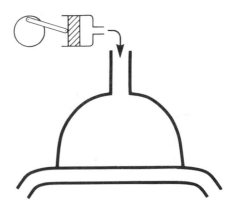

chapter **10**

Mechanical Ventilation

Artificial ventilation has become increasingly important in the management of patients with respiratory failure. Once used only as an emergency procedure in resuscitation or as a last resort in the treatment of the critically ill, it is now frequently employed to tide a patient over a respiratory crisis. Mechanical ventilation is a complex and technical subject and this discussion is limited to the physiological principles of its use, benefits, and hazards.

INTUBATION AND TRACHEOSTOMY

Most ventilators require a port for connection to the lung airway. An exception is the tank type of ventilator (see below), which is now rarely used. The connection is made by means of an endotracheal or tracheostomy tube. These are provided with an inflatable cuff at the end to give an airtight seal. Endotracheal tubes can be inserted via the nose or mouth.

These tubes have additional functions besides providing a connection for ventilators. They facilitate the removal of secretions by suction
188

catheter, a serious problem in many patients with respiratory failure. Retained secretions are particularly troublesome in patients who are obtunded, who have a suppressed cough reflex, or in whom the secretions are particularly copious or viscid. In addition, a tracheostomy may be necessary to bypass upper airway obstruction caused, for example by allergic edema or a laryngeal tumor. Also, the tube may prevent the aspiration of blood or vomitus from the pharynx into the lung.

The decision to intubate and ventilate a patient should not be lightly undertaken, since it is a major intervention requiring a substantial investment of personnel and equipment, with many possible hazards. On the other hand, patients are frequently intubated too late in the course of respiratory failure. The precise timing depends on such factors as the nature of the underlying disease process, the rapidity of the progress of hypoxemia and hypercapnia, and the age and general condition of the patient.

There are several complications associated with the use of endotracheal and tracheostomy tubes. Sudden occlusion by kinking or plugging may occur, especially if there is bleeding in the lower airway. Ulceration of the larynx or the trachea is sometimes seen. This is particularly likely if the inflated cuff exerts undue pressure on the mucosa; the subsequent scarring can result in tracheal stenosis. The use of large-volume, low-pressure cuffs has reduced the incidence of this problem. Also, care must be taken with the placement of an endotracheal tube. For example, if the cuff is inflated when the tube is in the right main bronchus, atelectasis of the left lung may ensue.

TYPES OF VENTILATORS

Constant-Volume Ventilators

Examples of these are the Bennet MA-2 and Siemens ventilators. They deliver a preset volume of gas to the patient, usually by means of a motor-driven piston in a cylinder (Figure 10.1) or a motor-driven bellows. The stroke and frequency of the pump can be adjusted to give the required ventilation; in some machines the ratio of inspiratory to expiratory time can be controlled by a special switching mechanism. Valves ensure that the patient is only connected to the pump during the inspiratory stroke. However, in some ventilators, expiration can be assisted by a small negative pressure developed by a Venturi device.

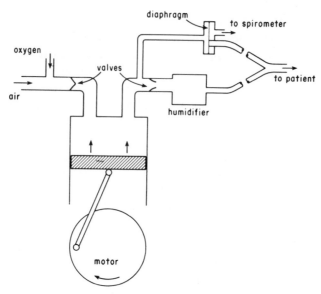

Figure 10.1. Example of a constant-volume ventilator (schematic). In practice the stroke volume and frequency can be regulated. During the expiratory phase, as the piston descends, the diaphragm is deflected to the left by the reduced pressure in the cylinder, allowing the patient to exhale through the spirometer.

Oxygen can be added to the inspired air as required, and a humidifier is included in the circuit.

Constant-volume ventilators are robust, dependable machines which are suitable for long-term ventilation. They are used extensively in anesthesia. They have the advantage that a known volume (or nearly so) is delivered to the patient in spite of changes in the elastic properties of the lung or chest wall or increases in airway resistance. A disadvantage is that high pressures can be developed; however, in practice, a safety blow-off valve prevents pressures from reaching dangerous levels. Estimating the patient's ventilation from the stroke volume and frequency of the pump may lead to important errors because of the compressibility of the gas and leaks, and it is better to measure the expired ventilation with a spirometer.

Constant-Pressure Ventilators

Examples of these are the Bennett PR-2 and Bird ventilators. They deliver gas at a preset pressure. They do not require electrical power but instead work off a source of compressed gas having a pressure of at least 50 pounds/square inch.

The principle of such a ventilator (Bird) is shown in Figure 10.2. The device consists essentially of two chambers known as the ambient and pressure chambers, separated by a diaphragm and sliding valve. During inspiration, shown in Figure 10.2A, the sliding valve is held to the right by the magnet X and gas enters the pressure chamber. When the preset pressure is reached, the diaphragm is distorted by the pressure across it and forces the valve to the left, thus cutting off the supply of gas (Figure 10.2B). The resulting change in pressure activates a valve in the line near the patient (not shown in Figure 10.2), expiration occurs, and the cycle is repeated.

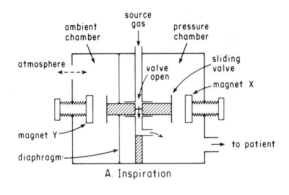

A. Inspiration

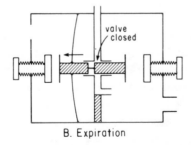

B. Expiration

Figure 10.2. Principle of a constant-pressure ventilator (schematic). In (A) the sliding valve is to the right and gas enters the pressure chamber and is delivered to the patient. When a preset pressure is reached, the diaphragm moves the valve to the left (B), thus cutting off the gas supply, and the patient exhales. (See text for further details.)

There are several additions to this basic operation. By adjustment of the position of magnet Y, the sliding valve can be held to the left in the exhalation position until the patient makes a small inspiratory effort. The reduced pressure then moves the diaphragm and valve to the right, thus delivering an inspiration to the patient. In this way the ventilator can assist the breathing of a patient in whom this is depressed. Inspiratory flow rate can be controlled by a needle valve in the line to the gas supply and appropriate mixtures of oxygen and air can be delivered. A nebulizer is included in the circuit. In some models, expiration of the patient can be assisted by negative pressure developed by a Venturi device.

Constant-pressure ventilators are versatile, small, and relatively inexpensive machines. Their chief disadvantage is that the volume of gas they deliver is altered by changes in the compliance of the lung or chest wall. Also, an increase in airway resistance may decrease the ventilation because there may be insufficient time for equilibration of pressure to occur between the machine and the alveoli. Expired volume should therefore be monitored, and this is difficult with some ventilators. Another disadvantage of some constant pressure ventilators is that the inspired oxygen concentration varies with the inspiratory flow rate.

Tank Ventilators

The ventilators we have discussed up to this point are called positive-pressure ventilators because they expand the lung by delivering positive pressure to the airway. By contrast, tank respirators deliver negative pressure (less than atmospheric) to the outside of the chest and rest of the body, excluding the head (Figure 10.3). They consist of a rigid box ("iron lung") connected to a large volume, low pressure pump which controls the respiratory cycle. The box is often hinged along the middle so that it can be opened to allow nursing care.

Tank ventilators are no longer used in the treatment of acute respiratory failure because they limit access to the patient and they are bulky and inconvenient. They were employed extensively to ventilate patients with bulbar poliomyelitis and they are still occasionally useful for patients with chronic neuromuscular disease who need to be ventilated for months or years. A modification of the tank ventilator is the cuirass, which fits over the thorax and abdomen and also

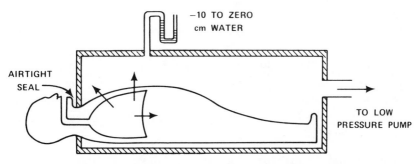

Figure 10.3. Tank respirator (schematic). The rigid box is connected to a large-volume, low pressure pump which swings the pressure from about 0 to −10 cm water.

generates negative pressure. It is usually reserved for patients who have partially recovered from neuromuscular respiratory failure.

Patient-Cycled Ventilators

In these ventilators the inspiratory phase can be triggered by the patient as he makes an inspiratory effort. The term "assisted ventilation" is sometimes given to this mode of operation. An example is the Bird ventilator of Figure 10.2, and generally the constant-pressure machines have this capability. These ventilators are particularly useful in the treatment of patients who are recovering from respiratory failure and who are being weaned from a period of controlled ventilation.

PATTERNS OF VENTILATION

Intermittent Positive Pressure Ventilation (IPPV)

This is sometimes called intermittent positive pressure breathing (IPPB) and is the common pattern in which the lung is expanded by the application of positive pressure to the airway and allowed to deflate passively to FRC. With modern ventilators the variables which can be controlled include the tidal volume, respiratory frequency, duration of inspiration versus expiration, and the inspiratory flow rate.

In patients with airway obstruction there is an advantage in prolonging the inspiratory time so that regions of the lung with long time constants have time to fill.* This can be done by reducing the respi-

---

* See J. B. West: *Respiratory Physiology—The Essentials*, ed. 3, p. 155. Baltimore, Williams & Wilkins, 1985.

ratory frequency and increasing the inspiratory versus expiratory time. On the other hand, a prolonged positive airway pressure may impede venous return to the thorax (see below), and therefore a compromise must be sought. Generally a relatively low frequency and an expiratory time greater than inspiratory time are selected, but each patient requires individual attention. In a few patients a small negative pressure is applied to the airway during expiration to reduce mean intrathoracic pressure.

Positive End-Expiratory Pressure (PEEP)

In patients with the adult respiratory distress syndrome, considerable improvement in the arterial P_{O_2} can often be obtained by maintaining a small positive airway pressure at the end of expiration. Values as low as 5 cm water are often beneficial, but pressures as high as 20 cm water or more are sometimes used. Special valves are available to provide the pressure, or the end of the expiratory line from the patient can simply be placed the appropriate distance under water. A secondary gain from PEEP is that is may allow the inspired oxygen concentration to be decreased, thus lessening the risk of oxygen toxicity.

Several mechanisms are probably responsible for the increase in arterial P_{O_2} resulting from PEEP. The positive pressure increases the FRC, which is typically very small in these patients because of the increased elastic recoil of the lung (see page 166). The low lung volume causes airway closure and intermittent ventilation (or none at all) of some areas, especially in the dependent regions (Figure 3.5), and absorption atelectasis ensues (Figure 9.6). PEEP tends to reverse these changes. Patients with edema in their airways also benefit, probably because the fluid is moved into small peripheral airways or alveoli, allowing some regions of the lung to be reventilated.

Figure 10.4 shows the effects of PEEP in a patient with the adult respiratory distress syndrome (45). Note that the level of PEEP was progressively increased from 0 to 16 cm H_2O and this caused the shunt to fall from 43.8 to 14.2% of the cardiac output. A small amount of blood flow to poorly ventilated alveoli remained. The increase in PEEP also caused the dead space to increase from 36.3 to 49.8% of the tidal volume. This can be explained partly by the increase in volume of the lung and consequent increased radial traction on the airways, and also probably compression of the capillaries by the increased alveolar pressure. This is discussed further on page 198.

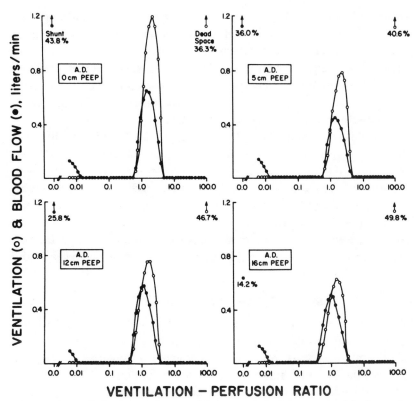

Figure 10.4. Reduction of shunt and increase of dead space caused by increasing levels of PEEP in a patient with the adult respiratory distress syndrome. Note that as the PEEP was progressively increased from 0 to 16 cm H_2O, the shunt decreased from 43.8 to 14.2% of the cardiac output, and the dead space increased from 36.3 to 49.8% of the tidal volume. (From D. R. Dantzker, C. J. Brook, P. DeHart, J. P. Lynch, and J. G. Weg: Ventilation-perfusion distributions in the adult respiratory distress syndrome. *Am. Rev. Respir. Dis.* 120:1039–1052, 1979 (45).)

Occasionally the addition of PEEP reduces rather than increases the arterial P_{O_2}. Possible mechanisms include 1) a substantial fall in cardiac output which reduces the P_{O_2} of mixed venous blood and therefore the arterial P_{O_2}, 2) reduced ventilation of well-perfused regions (because of increasing dead space and ventilation to poorly perfused regions), and 3) diversion of blood flow away from ventilated to unventilated regions by the raised airway pressure. This deleterious effect of PEEP on the arterial P_{O_2} is fortunately seldom seen.

PEEP tends to reduce cardiac output by impeding venous return to the thorax, especially if the circulating blood volume has been depleted by hemorrhage or shock. Accordingly, its value should not be gauged by its effect on the arterial P_{O_2} alone but in terms of the total amount of oxygen delivered to the tissues. The product of the arterial oxygen content and the cardiac output is a useful index, since changes in this alter the P_{O_2} of mixed venous blood and therefore the P_{O_2} of many tissues. Some physicians use the level of the P_{O_2} in mixed venous blood as a guide to the optimal level of PEEP.

However, in some extremely ill patients, the P_{O_2} of mixed venous blood can be misleading. It has been shown that under some conditions, the application of PEEP causes a reduction in overall oxygen consumption of the patient (46). Although this raises the oxygen content and P_{O_2} of mixed venous blood (see equation on page 178) this is not beneficial to the patient. Apparently the oxygen consumption falls because the perfusion of some tissues is so marginal that if their blood flow is further decreased, they are unable to take up oxygen, and presumably slowly die.

Continuous Positive Airway Pressure (CPAP)

Some patients who are being weaned from a ventilator breathe spontaneously but are still intubated. Such patients may benefit from a small positive pressure applied continuously to the airway. The pressure can be obtained by passing gas at a high flow rate through a T piece attached to the endotracheal tube and thence to a water bottle. The improvement in oxygenation results from the same mechanisms as for PEEP. A form of CPAP had been used successfully in the treatment of the infant respiratory distress syndrome.

Intermittent Mandatory Ventilation (IMV)

This is a modification of IPPV (see above) in which a large tidal volume is given at relatively infrequent intervals to an intubated patient who is breathing spontaneously. It is often combined with PEEP or CPAP. This pattern may be useful in weaning a patient from a ventilator.

High Frequency Ventilation

Recent experimental work has shown that it is possible to maintain normal blood gases by using very high frequency (about 20 cycles/sec) positive-pressure ventilation with very low stroke volumes (50–100 ml). The lung is vibrated rather than expanded in the conventional way, and the transport of the gas is believed to be by some kind of facilitated diffusion. It is too early to say how useful this will be in clinical practice, but it looks promising for some patients with the infant respiratory distress syndrome.

PHYSIOLOGICAL EFFECTS OF MECHANICAL VENTILATION

Reduction of Arterial P_{CO_2}

In general, mechanical ventilation is used to increase ventilation and improve pulmonary gas exchange in lungs in which it is grossly defective. This may be either because the patient is not able to breathe spontaneously, as in neuromuscular disease, or because the lung itself is severely diseased, as in the adult respiratory distress syndrome. Frequently, mechanical ventilation is begun because the arterial P_{CO_2} is rising or already elevated, and it is usually very effective at keeping this in check or reducing it. In patients with airway obstruction in whom the oxygen cost of breathing is very high, mechanical ventilation may appreciably reduce the oxygen uptake and CO_2 output, thus contributing to the fall in arterial P_{CO_2}.

The relationship between the arterial P_{CO_2} and the alveolar ventilation in normal lungs is given by the familiar equation:

$$P_{CO_2} = \frac{\dot{V}_{CO_2}}{\dot{V}_A} \cdot K$$

where K is a constant. In diseased lungs the denominator $\dot{V}_A$ in this equation is less than the ventilation going to the alveoli because of alveolar dead space, that is, unperfused alveoli or those with high ventilation-perfusion ratios (see page 36). For this reason the denominator is sometimes referred to as the "effective alveolar ventilation."

Mechanical ventilation frequently increases both the alveolar and anatomical dead spaces. As a consequence, the effective alveolar ventilation is not increased as much as the total ventilation. This is particularly likely if high pressures are applied to the airway. This can be seen in the example shown in Figure 10.4. As the level of PEEP was increased from 0 to 16 cm H_2O in this patient with the adult respiratory distress syndrome, the dead space increased from 36.3 to 49.8%. In some patients, high levels of PEEP also result in the appearance of lung units with high ventilation-perfusion ratios which cause a shoulder to form on the right of the ventilation distribution curve. This did not occur in the example shown. Occasionally a large physiological dead space is seen with IPPV even in the absence of PEEP. An example is shown in Figure 8.3.

There are several reasons why positive-pressure ventilation increases dead space. First, lung volume is usually raised, especially when PEEP is added, and the resulting radial traction on the airways increases the anatomical dead space. Next, the raised airway pressure tends to divert blood flow away from ventilated regions, thus causing areas of high ventilation-perfusion ratio or even unperfused areas (Figure 10.4). This is particularly likely to happen in the uppermost regions of the lung where the pulmonary artery pressure is relatively low because of the hydrostatic effect.* Indeed, if the pressure in the capillaries falls below airway pressure, the capillaries may collapse completely, resulting in unperfused lung (Figure 10.5) (47). This is encouraged by two factors: 1) the abnormally high airway pressure, and 2) the reduced venous return and consequent hypoperfusion of the lung. The latter is particularly likely to occur if there is a reduced circulating blood volume (see below).

The tendency for the arterial P_{CO_2} to rise as a result of the increased dead space can be countered by resetting the ventilator to increase the total ventilation. Nevertheless, it is important to remember that an increase in mean airway pressure can cause a substantial rise in dead space, although the increased pressure may be necessary to combat the shunt and resulting hypoxemia (Figure 10.4).

In practice, many patients who are mechanically ventilated develop an abnormally low arterial P_{CO_2} because they are overventilated. This results in a respiratory alkalosis which frequently coexists with a metabolic acidosis because of the hypoxemia and impaired peripheral circulation. An unduly low arterial P_{CO_2} should be avoided because it reduces cerebral blood flow and therefore contributes to cerebral hypoxia.

Another hazard of overventilation in patients with CO_2 retention is a low serum potassium, which predisposes to abnormal heart rhythms. The reason for this is that when CO_2 is retained, potassium moves out of the cells into the plasma and is excreted by the kidney. If the P_{CO_2}

---

* See J. B. West: *Respiratory Physiology—The Essentials*, ed. 3, p. 40. Baltimore, Williams & Wilkins, 1985.

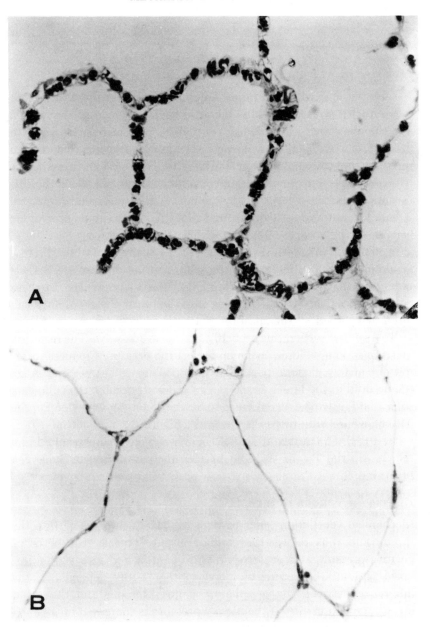

Figure 10.5. Effect of raised airway pressure on the histological appearance of pulmonary capillaries. (A) Normal appearance. (B) Collapse of capillaries when alveolar pressure is raised above capillary pressure. (From J. B. Glazier, J. M. B. Hughes, J. E. Maloney, and J. B. West: Measurements of capillary dimensions and blood volume in rapidly frozen lungs. *J. Appl. Physiol.* 26:65–76, 1969 (47).)

is then rapidly reduced, the potassium moves back into the cells, thus depleting the plasma.

Increase in Arterial P_{O_2}

In some patients with respiratory failure, for example, those with adult respiratory distress syndrome, the arterial P_{CO_2} is typically not raised and the objective of mechanical ventilation is to increase the P_{O_2}. In practice, such patients are always ventilated with enriched oxygen mixtures and the combination is usually very effective in relieving the hypoxemia. The inspired oxygen concentration should ideally be sufficient to raise the arterial P_{O_2} to the normal range, for example above 80 mm Hg, but unduly high inspired concentrations should be avoided because of the hazards of oxygen toxicity and atelectasis.

In some patients with severe forms of the adult respiratory distress syndrome, intermittent positive pressure ventilation with 100% O_2 is not successful in raising the arterial P_{O_2} above 70 mm Hg. In these circumstances the life-threatening hypoxemia of these patients can often be relieved by the addition of PEEP of 5–20 cm water (Figure 10.4). As noted earlier, this probably acts in several ways. The resulting increase in lung volume opens up atelectatic areas and reduces intermittent airway closure, particularly in the dependent regions. Also, edema fluid in the larger airways is moved peripherally, thus allowing some previously obstructed areas to be ventilated. As an example, the patient whose lung biopsy is shown in Figure 8.2 was put on 10 cm water PEEP on the day after the biopsy was taken. This resulted in a rise in arterial P_{O_2} of from 80 to 130 mm Hg during 80% oxygen breathing.

Effects on Venous Return

Mechanical ventilation tends to impede the return of blood into the thorax and thus reduce the cardiac output. This is true both for positive-pressure and negative-pressure ventilation. In a supine, relaxed patient, the return of blood to the thorax depends on the difference between the peripheral venous pressure and the mean intrathoracic pressure. If the airway pressure is increased by a ventilator, mean intrathoracic pressure rises and venous return is impeded (Figure 10.6) (48). Even if airway pressure remains atmospheric, as in a tank respirator (Figure 10.3), venous return tends to fall because the

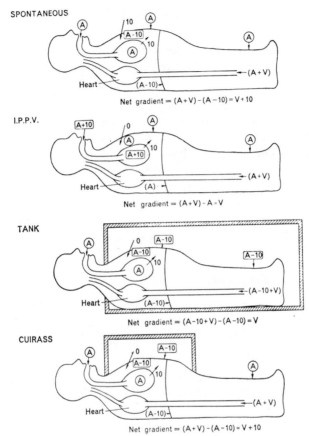

Figure 10.6. Effect of mechanical ventilation on venous return. The diagram shows typical pressures at the end of inspiration. A, atmospheric pressure; V, peripheral venous pressure (mm Hg). The pressure across the chest wall is indicated by the *downward arrow*; this is zero (except for spontaneous respiration), because at this lung volume the chest wall is in its relaxed position. Transpulmonary pressure is represented by the *upward arrow*. Note that the pressure gradient responsible for venous return is reduced by IPPV and tank respirators but not by the cuirass type. (From M. K. Sykes, M. W. McNicol, and E. J. M. Campbell: *Respiratory Failure*, ed. 2. Oxford, Blackwell, 1976 (48).)

peripheral venous pressure is reduced by the negative pressure. Only in the cuirass respirator is venous return virtually unaffected.

The effects of positive-pressure ventilation on venous return depend on the magnitude and duration of the inspiratory pressure and, particularly, the addition of PEEP. The ideal pattern from this standpoint is a short inspiratory phase of relatively low pressure followed by a long expiratory phase and zero (or slightly negative) end-expiratory pressure. However, such a pattern encourages a low lung volume and consequent hypoxemia, and a compromise is generally necessary.

An important determinant of venous return is the magnitude of the circulating blood volume. If this is reduced, for example, by hemorrhage or shock, positive-pressure ventilation often causes a marked fall in cardiac output. Systemic hypotension may ensue. It is therefore important to correct any volume depletion by appropriate fluid replacement. The central venous pressure is often monitored as a guide to this but should be interpreted in the light of the increased airway pressure. Positive airway pressure itself raises central venous pressure. An additional factor often contributing to the fall in cardiac output during mechanical ventilation is hypocapnia caused by overventilation.

Miscellaneous Hazards

Mechanical problems are a constant hazard. They include power failure, broken connections, and kinking of tubes. Apnea alarms are available to warn of these dangers, but skilled care by the intensive care team is essential.

Pneumothorax can occur, especially if PEEP and/or unusually large tidal volumes are used. *Interstitial emphysema* may develop if the lung is overdistended. The air escapes from ruptured alveoli, tracks along the perivascular and peribronchial interstitium (Figure 6.1), and may enter the mediastinum and the subcutaneous tissue of the neck.

Pulmonary infection is a danger if the equipment is not scrupulously clean. Crusting of the large airways occurs unless the gas is efficiently humidified. *Cardiac arrhythmias* may be caused by rapid swings in pH and hypoxemia. There is also an increased incidence of *gastrointestinal bleeding* in these patients.

Appendix

SYMBOLS

Primary

C Concentration of gas in blood
F Fractional concentration in dry gas
P Pressure or partial pressure
Q Volume of blood
$\dot{Q}$ Volume of blood per unit time
R Respiratory exchange ratio
S Saturation of hemoglobin with O_2
V Volume of gas
$\dot{V}$ Volume of gas per unit time

Secondary Symbols for Gas Phase

A Alveolar
B Barometric
D Dead Space
E Expired
I Inspired
L Lung
T Tidal

Secondary Symbols for Blood Phase

a arterial
c capillary
c' end-capillary
i ideal
v venous
$\bar{v}$ mixed venous

Examples

O_2 concentration in arterial blood Ca_{O_2}
Fractional concentration of N_2 in expired gas FE_{N_2}
Partial pressure of O_2 in mixed venous blood $P\bar{v}_{O_2}$

UNITS

Traditional metric units have been used in this book. Pressures are given in mm Hg; the torr is an almost identical unit.

In Europe, SI (Système Internationale) units are now commonly used. Most of these are familiar, but the kilopascal, the new unit of pressure, is confusing at first. One kilopascal = 7.5 mm Hg.

Conversion of Gas Volumes to BTPS*

Lung volumes including FEV and FVC are conventionally expressed at body temperature (37° C), ambient pressure, and saturated with water vapor (BTPS). To convert volumes measured in a spirometer at ambient temperature (t), pressure, saturated (ATPS) to BTPS, multiply by

$$\frac{310}{273 + t} \cdot \frac{P_B - P_{H_2O}(t)}{P_B - 47}$$

In practice, tables are available for this conversion (4).

NORMAL VALUES

Normal Values for Lung Function Tests

Normal values depend on age, sex, height, weight, and ethnic origin. This is a complex subject, and for a detailed discussion the reader is referred to Chapter 14 of J. E. Cotes: *Lung Function* (4th ed.), Oxford: Blackwell, 1979. Normal values for the commonly used tests are shown in Table A-1. Reference 49 contains another useful discussion of normal values.

As an example of the use of table A-1, suppose we wish to know whether an $FEV_{1.0}$ of 3.2 liters in a 25-year-old man of height 1.83 m is abnormally low. From the table, the predicted value is:

$$(3.7 \times 1.83) - (0.028 \times 25) - 1.59 = 4.48 \text{ liters}$$

Since from the table the SD is 0.52 liters, the predicted value −1.65 SD = 3.62 liters. Therefore, the measured value of 3.2 liters is very likely to be abnormally low. The value of 1.65 rather than 2 SD is

* For more details see J. B. West: *Respiratory Physiology—The Essentials*, ed. 3, p. 162. Baltimore, Williams & Wilkins, 1985.

Table A-1. Regression relationships for predicting indices of function from age (yr), height (m) and weight (kg) in healthy adults of European descent; gas volumes are expressed as BTPS (body temperature and pressure, saturated with water vapor); for main sources of data, see Cotes (4), Tables 14.11 and 14.12; the values for the single breath N_2 test and the closing volume are from References 50 and 51, respectively.

Index	Sex	Regression Coefficients			Constant Term	SD
		Height	Age	Weight		
Total lung capacity (liters)	M	7.8			−7.3	0.87
	F	7.46	−0.013		−6.42	0.51
Vital capacity (liters)	M	5.20	−0.022		−3.60	0.58
	F	4.66	−0.029		−2.88	0.44
Residual volume (liters)	M	2.7	+0.017		−3.45	0.39
	F	2.8	+0.016		−3.54	0.31
FRC (liters)	M	3.2			−2.94	0.63
	F	6.60		−0.03	−5.76	0.43
$FEV_{1.0}$ (liters)	M	3.7	−0.028		−1.59	0.52
	F	3.29	−0.029		−1.42	0.36
$(FEV_{1.0}/FVC) \times 100$ (%)	M		−0.373		+91.8	7.19
	F		−0.222		+86.5	6.2
$FEF_{25-75\%}$ (liters/sec)	M		−0.057		+6.38	1.09
	F		−0.063		+6.14	0.77
Single breath N_2 test (% liter)	M		+0.010		+0.710	0.43
	F <60 yr		+0.009		+1.036	0.57
Closing volume/VC (%)	M		+0.357		+0.562	4.15
	F		+0.293		+2.812	4.90
Arterial P_{O_2} (mm Hg)			−0.24		+104	7.9
Arterial P_{CO_2} (mm Hg)					37–43	
Arterial pH					7.35–7.45	
D_{CO} (ml/min/mm Hg)	M	32.6	−0.20		−17.61	5.1
	F	21.2	−0.16		−2.66	3.6
Airway resistance (cm H_2O/liter/sec)					0.5–2.0	
Lung compliance (liter/ cm H_2O)					0.09–0.40	

used because we are asking the question: Is the observed FEV abnormally low (as opposed to simply abnormal)? However, it should be noted that the use of the reported SD involves many assumptions, and care should be taken not to imply a spurious precision (4).

References

1. FERRIS, B. G. Epidemiology standardization project. *Am. Rev. Respir. Dis. Suppl.* 118:1–120, 1978.
2. LEUALLEN, E. C., AND W. S. FOWLER. Maximal midexpiratory flow. *Am. Rev. Tuberculosis* 72:783–800, 1955.
3. DOSMAN, J., F. BODE, J. URBANETTI, R. MARTIN, AND P. T. MACKLEM. The use of a helium-oxygen mixture during maximum expiratory flow to demonstrate obstruction in small airways in smokers. *J. Clin. Invest.* 55:1090–1099, 1975.
4. COTES, J. E. *Lung Function* (4th ed.). Oxford: Blackwell, 1979.
5. HINSON, K. F. W. Diffuse pulmonary fibrosis. *Hum. Pathol.* 1:275–288, 1970.
6. RILEY, R. L., AND A. COURNAND. "Ideal" alveolar air and the analysis of ventilation-perfusion relationships in the lung. *J. Appl. Physiol.* 1:825–847, 1949.
7. WAGNER, P. D., R. B. LARAVUSO, R. R. UHL, AND J. B. WEST. Continuous distributions of ventilation-perfusion ratios in normal subjects breathing air and 100% O_2. *J. Clin Invest.* 54:54–68, 1974.
8. FLENLEY, D. C. Another non-logarithmic acid-base diagram? *Lancet* 1:961–965, 1971.
9. BATES, D. V., P. T. MACKLEM, AND R. V. CHRISTIE. *Respiratory Function in Disease* (2nd ed.). Philadelphia: W. B. Saunders, 1971.
10. NADEL, J. A., AND J. H. COMROE, JR. Acute effects of inhalation of cigarette smoke on airway conductance. *J. Appl. Physiol.* 16:713–716, 1961.
11. READ, D. J. C. A clinical method for assessing the ventilatory response to carbon dioxide. *Australas. Ann. Med.* 16:20–32, 1967.
12. WHITELAW, W. A., J.-P. DERENNE, AND J. MILIC-EMILI. Occlusion pressure as a measure of respiratory center output in conscious man. *Resp. Physiol.* 23:181–199, 1975.
13. LANE, D. J., AND J. B. L. HOWELL. Relationship between sensitivity to carbon dioxide and clinical features in patients with chronic airways obstruction. *Thorax* 25:150–159, 1970.
14. JONES, N. L. Exercise testing in pulmonary evaluation. *N. Engl. J. Med.* 293:541–544, 647–650, 1975.
15. JONES, N. L., E. J. M. CAMPBELL, R. H. T. EDWARDS, AND D. G. ROBERTSON. *Clinical Exercise Testing.* Philadelphia: W. B. Saunders, 1975.
16. HEARD, B. E. *Pathology of Chronic Bronchitis and Emphysema.* London: Churchill, 1969.
17. MITTMAN, C. (Ed.). *Pulmonary Emphysema and Proteolysis.* New York: Academic Press, 1972.

18. THURLBECK, W. M. *Chronic Airflow Obstruction in Lung Disease.* Philadelphia: W. B. Saunders, 1976.
19. BURROWS, B., C. M. FLETCHER, B. E. HEARD, N. L. JONES, AND J. S. WOOTLIFF. The emphysematous and bronchial types of chronic airways obstruction. *Lancet* 1:830–835, 1966.
20. COLEBATCH, H. J. H., K. E. FINUCANE, AND M. M. SMITH. Pulmonary conductance and elastic recoil relationships in asthma and emphysema. *J. Appl. Physiol.* 34:143–153, 1973.
21. WAGNER, P. D., D. R. DANTZKER, R. DUECK, J. L. CLAUSEN, AND J. B. WEST. Ventilation-perfusion inequality in chronic pulmonary disease. *J. Clin. Invest.* 59:203–206, 1977.
22. MACKLEM, P. T. Airway obstruction and collateral ventilation. *Physiol. Rev.* 368–436, 1971.
23. CHERNIACK, R. M., L. CHERNIACK, AND A. NAIMARK. *Respiration in Health and Disease* (2nd ed.). Philadelphia, W. B. Saunders, 1972.
24. WEISS, E. B., M. S. SEGAL, AND M. STEIN. *Bronchial Asthma. Mechanisms and Therapeutics* (2nd ed.) Boston: Little, Brown, 1985.
25. KAY, A. B., K. F. AUSTEN, AND L. M. LICHTENSTEIN (Eds.). *Asthma, Physiology, Immunopharmacology and Treatment.* New York: Academic Press, 1984.
26. WEIBEL, E. R. Morphological basis of alveolar-capillary gas exchange. *Physiol. Rev.* 53:419–495, 1973.
27. WEIBEL, E. R., AND J. GIL. Structure-function relationships at the alveolar level. In *Bioengineering Aspects of the Lung.* Edited by J. B. West. New York: Marcel Dekker, 1977.
28. GRACEY, D. R., M. B. DIVERTIE, AND A. L. BROWN, JR. Alveolar-capillary membrane in idiopathic interstitial pulmonary fibrosis. Electron microscopic study of 14 cases. *Am. Rev. Respir. Dis.* 98:16–21, 1968.
29. HAMMAN, L., AND A. R. RICH. Acute diffuse interstitial fibrosis of the lungs. *Bull. Johns Hopkins Hosp.* 74:177–212, 1944.
30. WEST J. B. Ventilation-perfusion relationships. *Am. Rev. Respir. Dis.* 116:919–943, 1977.
31. STAUB, N. C. Pulmonary edema. *Physiol. Rev.* 54:679–811, 1974.
32. STAUB, N. C. The pathophysiology of pulmonary edema. *Hum. Pathol.* 1:419–432, 1970.
33. ROBIN, E. D., C. E. CROSS, AND R. ZELIS. Pulmonary edema. *N. Engl. J. Med.* 288:239–246, 292–304, 1973.
34. SEVERINGHAUS, J. W., E. W. SWENSON, T. N. FINLEY, M. T. LATEGOLA, AND J. WILLIAMS. Unilateral hypoventilation produced in dogs by occluding one pulmonary artery. *J. Appl. Physiol.* 16:53–60, 1961.
35. DANTZKER, D. R., P. D. WAGNER, V. W. TORNABENE, N. P. ALZARAKI, AND J. B. WEST. Gas exchange after pulmonary thromboembolization in dogs. *Circ. Res.* 42:92–103, 1978.
36. D'ALONZO G. E., J. S. BOWER, P. DeHART, AND D. R. DANTZKER. The mechanisms of abnormal gas exchange in acute massive pulmonary embolism. *Am. Rev. Respir. Dis.* 128:170–172, 1983.
37. NEWHOUSE, M., J. SANCHIS, AND J. BIENENSTOCK. Lung defense mechanisms. *N. Engl. J. Med.* 295:990–998, 1045–1052, 1976.
38. HEPPLESTON, A. G., AND J. G. LEOPOLD. Chronic pulmonary emphysema: anatomy and pathogenesis. *Am. J. Med.* 31:279–291, 1961.

39. ULMER, W. T., AND G. REICHEL. Functional impairment in coal worker's pneumoconiosis. *Ann. N.Y. Acad. Sci.* 200:405–412, 1972.
40. HOPEWELL, P. C., AND J. F. MURRAY. The adult respiratory distress syndrome. *Annu. Rev. Med.* 27:343–356, 1976.
41. LAMY, M., R. J. FALLAT, E. KOENIGER, H.-P. DIETRICH, J. L. RATLIFF, R. C. EBERHART, H. J. TUCKER, AND J. D. HILL. Pathologic features and mechanisms of hypoxemia in adult respiratory syndrome. *Am. Rev. Respir. Dis.* 114:267–284, 1976.
42. FARRELL, P. M., AND M. E. AVERY. Hyaline membrane disease. *Am. Rev. Respir. Dis.* 111:657–688, 1975.
43. WEST, J. B., AND P. D. WAGNER. Pulmonary gas exchange. In *Bioengineering Aspects of The Lung.* Edited by J. B. West. New York: Marcel Dekker, 1977.
44. KAPANCI, U., E. R. WEIBEL, H. P. KAPLAN, AND F. R. ROBINSON. Pathogenesis and reversibility of the pulmonary lesions of oxygen toxicity in monkeys. *Lab. Invest.* 20:101–118, 1969.
45. DANTZKER, D. R., C. J. BROOK, P. DeHART, J. P. LYNCH, AND J. G. WEG. Ventilation-perfusion distributions in the adult respiratory distress syndrome. *Am. Rev. Respir. Dis.* 120:1039–1052, 1979.
46. DANEK, S. J., J. P. LYNCH, J. G. WEG, AND D. R. DANTZKER. The dependence of the oxygen uptake on oxygen delivery in the adult respiratory distress syndrome. *Am. Rev. Respir. Dis.* 122:387–395, 1980.
47. GLAZIER, J. B., J. M. B. HUGHES, J. E. MALONEY, AND J. B. WEST. Measurements of capillary dimensions and blood volume in rapidly frozen lungs. *J. Appl. Physiol.* 26:65–76, 1969.
48. SYKES, M. K., M. W. McNICOL, AND E. J. M. CAMPBELL. *Respiratory Failure* (2nd ed.). Oxford: Blackwell, 1976.
49. CLAUSEN, J. (Ed.). *Pulmonary Function Testing Guidelines and Controversies.* New York: Academic Press, 1982.
50. BUIST, A. S., AND B. J. ROSS. Quantitative analysis of the alveolar plateau in the diagnosis of airway obstruction. *Am. Rev. Respir. Dis.* 108:1078–1087, 1973.
51. BUIST, A. S., AND B. J. ROSS. Predicted values for closing volume using a modified single breath test. *Am. Rev. Respir. Dis.* 107:744–752, 1973.

Further Reading

The list of references (page 206) provides additional information about some specific topics referred to in the text. Other sources of general interest are as follows.

Lung Function Tests and What They Mean

BATES, D. V., P. T. MACKLEM, AND R. V. CHRISTIE. *Respiratory Function in Disease* (2nd ed.). Philadelphia: W. B. Saunders, 1971.

BOUHUYS, A. *Breathing.* New York: Grune and Stratton, 1974.

CHERNIACK, R. M., L. CHERNIACK, AND A. NAIMARK. *Respiration in Health and Disease* (3rd ed.). Chicago, Year Book, 1983.

COTES, J. E. *Lung Function* (4th ed.). Oxford: Blackwell, 1979.

CUMMING, G., AND S. SEMPLE. *Disorders of the Respiratory System* (2nd ed.). St. Louis: Mosby, 1980.

FISHMAN, A. P. *Assessment of Pulmonary Function.* New York: McGraw Hill, 1980.

MURRAY, J. F. *The Normal Lung* (2nd ed.). Philadelphia: W. B. Saunders, 1986.

NUNN, J. F. *Applied Respiratory Physiology* (2nd ed.). New York: Appleton-Century-Crofts, 1977.

WEST, J. B. *Ventilation/Bloodflow and Gas Exchange* (4th ed.). Oxford: Blackwell, 1985.

Function of the Diseased Lung

Most of the books listed above. In addition:

BRAUNWALD, E. (Ed.). *Harrison's Principles of Internal Medicine* (11th ed.). New York: McGraw Hill, 1987.

CROFTON, J., AND A. DOUGLAS. *Respiratory Diseases* (3rd ed.). Oxford: Blackwell, 1981.

FRASER, R. G., AND J. A. P. PARÉ. *Diagnosis of Diseases of the Chest* (2nd ed.). Philadelphia: Saunders, 1977.

HEARD, B. E. *Pathology of Chronic Bronchitis and Emphysema.* London: Churchill, 1969.

MUIR, D. C. F. (Ed.). *Clinical Aspects of Inhaled Particles.* London: Heinemann, 1972.

NADEL, J. A., AND J. F. MURRAY. *Textbook of Pulmonary Disease.* Philadelphia: W. B. Saunders, 1987.

REID, L. *Pathology of Emphysema.* Chicago: Year Book, 1967.

SPENCER, H. *Pathology of The Lung* (4th ed.). New York: Pergamon, 1985.

THURLBECK, W. M. *Chronic Airflow Obstruction in Lung Disease.* Philadelphia: W. B. Saunders, 1976.

WEISS, E. B., M. S. SEGAL, AND M. STEIN. *Bronchial Asthma* (2nd ed.). Boston: Little, Brown, 1985.

Function of the Failing Lung

Appropriate sections of the books listed above. In addition:

EGAN, D. F. *Fundamentals of Respiratory Therapy* (4th ed.). St. Louis: Mosby, 1982.

HEDLEY-WHITE, J., G. E. BURGESS, III, T. W. FEELEY, AND H. G. MILLER. *Applied Physiology of Respiratory Care*. Boston: Little, Brown, 1976.

PONTOPPIDAN, H., B. FEFFIN, AND E. LOWENSTEIN. *Acute Respiratory Failure in the Adult*. Boston: Little, Brown, 1973.

SYKES, M. K., M. W. McNICOL, AND E. J. M. CAMPBELL. *Respiratory Failure* (2nd ed.). Oxford: Blackwell, 1976.

Questions

(For answers see page 220)

Note: when several possible answers are given, more than one may be correct.

CHAPTER 1

1. Define a) 1 sec forced expiratory volume, and b) forced expiratory flow.
2. Maximum flow rate during most of a forced expiration is normally limited by: a) turbulence in the trachea, b) rate of contraction of the respiratory muscles, c) action of the diaphragm, d) compression of the airways, e) abdominal muscles.
3. During most of a forced expiration, what pressure difference is responsible for the flow rate?
4. Which of the following factors may reduce the $FEV_{1.0}$ in a patient with chronic obstructive lung disease? a) excessive secretions in the airways, b) reduction in number of small airways, c) loss of radial traction on airways, d) loss of elastic recoil of lung, e) respiratory acidosis.
5. Which of the following factors may contribute to an abnormally high forced expiratory flow rate (in relation to lung volume) in a patient with advanced interstitial fibrosis? a) hypertrophy of abdominal muscles, b) increased lung elastic recoil, c) increased radial traction on the airways.
6. Which of the following results suggest an increased resistance of the peripheral small airways? a) reduced peak flow rate, b) low maximal flow rate at 10% VC, c) large increase in maximal flow rate at 50% VC when a helium-oxygen mixture is breathed.
7. In a patient with lung disease who has a reduced $FEF_{25-75\%}$ a plot of maximum expiratory flow rate against static elastic recoil pressure shows a normal relationship. This suggests: a) reduced elastic recoil but normal airways, b) obstructed airways and reduced elastic recoil, c) normal elastic recoil but diseased airways.
8. In a patient with mild lung disease, which of the following factors are likely to be responsible for an increased slope of phase 3 (alveolar plateau) in the single breath N_2 test? a) uneven time constants within the lung, b) series inequality of ventilation, c) airway closure in the dependent regions, d) cardiogenic oscillations.

9. The closing volume as determined from a single breath N_2 test: a) is most informative in patients with severe lung disease, b) is thought to reflect the state of small peripheral airways, c) is highly reproducible in normal subjects, d) normally increases with age.

10. After an upright normal subject takes a vital capacity breath of pure O_2 the N_2 concentration at the apex exceeds that at the base because: a) airway closure at the base delays filling of that region, b) airway resistance of lower zones is high, c) the ventilation-perfusion ratio is high at the apex, d) the apical alveoli expand less than those at the base.

CHAPTER 2

1. The oxygen electrode: a) is a sensitive pH meter, b) measures the EMF (voltage) developed by the O_2 in a sample of blood, c) measures the current flowing through a buffer of given P_{O_2}, d) consumes O_2.

2. In peripheral capillaries, more O_2 can be unloaded from blood at a given P_{O_2} when: a) blood temperature is reduced, b) P_{CO_2} is raised, c) blood pH is raised, d) concentration of 2,3-DPG in the red cells is raised.

3. A young man with normal lungs takes an overdose of barbiturate and hypoventilates. Which of the following will probably reach the value of 50 first (assume usual units)? a) arterial P_{O_2}, b) arterial O_2 saturation, c) arterial P_{CO_2}, d) plasma bicarbonate concentration.

4. In a patient with severe diffuse interstitial fibrosis of the lung, factors which are likely to contribute to the hypoxemia on exercise include: a) reduced alveolar ventilation, b) reduced time spent by the blood in the pulmonary capillaries, c) ventilation-perfusion inequality.

5. What is meant by the term ideal alveolar P_{O_2}?

6. What is the equation for deriving the physiological dead space from the arterial and mixed expired P_{CO_2}?

7. Why is a patient with $V_A/\dot{Q}$ inequality able to maintain a normal arterial P_{CO_2} but not P_{O_2} by increasing the ventilation to his alveoli?

8. A previously well patient takes an overdose of a narcotic drug and is brought to the emergency room, where the arterial P_{CO_2} is found to be 80 mm Hg. What value would you expect for the arterial pH?

9. A patient with chronic lung disease undergoes emergency surgery. Post-operatively the arterial P_{O_2}, P_{CO_2}, and pH are 50, 50 (mm Hg), and 7.20, respectively. What terms would best describe the probable acid-base status?

10. Which of the following factors probably contribute to the reduced diffusing capacity for CO in a patient with emphysema? a) loss of pulmonary capillaries, b) reduced elastic recoil, c) uneven distribution of ventilation, blood flow and diffusion properties, d) increased FRC.

CHAPTER 3

1. Which of the following typically results in an increased FRC? a) emphysema, b) attack of asthma, c) pulmonary sarcoidosis, d) pulmonary embolism, e) normal aging.

2. In a patient with bullous lung disease it was found that the FRC as determined in the body plethysmograph was much greater than that measured by helium dilution. Probable explanations include: a) some regions of the lung were very poorly ventilated, b) some regions were completely unventilated, c) some regions had a high blood flow in relation to lung volume.

3. In which of the following conditions is the elastic recoil of the lung typically increased? a) interstitial fibrosis, b) attack of asthma, c) emphysema, d) mitral stenosis, e) normal aging.

4. Which of the following factors may contribute to the increase in airway resistance in asthma? a) edema of airway walls, b) contraction of bronchial smooth muscle, c) abnormal secretions in the airway, d) increased alveolar P_{CO_2}.

5. Which of the following factors may contribute to the impaired ventilatory response to inhaled CO_2 in a patient with chronic obstructive lung disease? a) increased inspiratory work for a given ventilation, b) increased compliance of the chest wall, c) reduced neural output of the respiratory center, d) arterial hypoxemia.

6. During an exercise test in a patient with mitral stenosis is was found that the respiratory exchange ratio rapidly rose above 1 at a low level of exercise. What were the probable reasons?

7. The apex, compared with the base, of the upright lung has: a) less blood flow, b) less ventilation, c) smaller alveoli, d) smaller mechanical stresses, e) less tendency for closure of small airways.

CHAPTER 4

1. What is meant by the term "emphysema"?

2. What is the typical topographical distribution within the lung of: a) centrilobular emphysema, b) emphysema caused by α_1-antitrypsin deficiency, c) panlobular emphysema.

3. α_1-Antitrypsin deficiency: a) causes severe bronchitis with emphysema, b) results in emphysema at a relatively early age, c) is genetically determined, d) is common in heterozygotes for the Z gene, e) particularly affects the apices of the lung.

4. What is the Reid index of chronic bronchitis?

5. Patients with chronic obstructive lung disease of type A (as opposed to type B) tend to have: a) more cough productive of sputum, b) larger lung volumes, c) lower lung elastic recoil, d) more hypoxemia, 3) more hypercapnia, f) lower diffusing capacity, g) greater tendency to develop cor pulmonale.

6. In a patient with severe chronic bronchitis and emphysema, which of the following is likely to be normal? a) $FEV_{1.0}$, b) VC, c) $FEV_{1.0}/FVC$, d) $FEF_{25-75\%}$, e) $\dot{V}_{max_{50}\%}$, f) forced expiratory time.

7. If airway conductance (Y) is plotted against static transpulmonary pressure (X), what are the typical findings in patients with: a) pure emphysema, b) asthma?

8. What is the chief mechanism of hypoxemia in patients with chronic obstructive lung disease? a) hypoventilation, b) diffusion impairment, c) shunt, d) ventilation-perfusion inequality?

9. Factors responsible for the increased pulmonary artery pressure in patients with chronic obstructive lung disease include a) destruction of parts of the pulmonary capillary bed, b) hypoxic vasoconstriction in low $\dot{V}_A/\dot{Q}$ areas, c) polycythemia, d) smooth muscle hypertrophy in some small arteries, e) systemic hypoxemia.

10. Abnormal features of the bronchi in asthma include: a) hypertrophied smooth muscle, b) hypertrophy of mucous glands, c) edema of bronchial walls, d) mucous plugging of some airways, e) collapse because of destruction of surrounding parenchyma, f) hypertrophy of cilia.

11. Mediators responsible for the bronchoconstriction in asthma probably include: a) histamine, b) angiotensin, c) bradykinin, d) norepinephrine, e) SRS-A.

12. Administration of isoproterenol to a patient with asthma frequently reduces the arterial P_{O_2}. The probable reason is: a) increase in cardiac output, b) selective bronchodilation in high $\dot{V}_A/\dot{Q}$ areas, c) selective vasodilation in low $\dot{V}_A/\dot{Q}$ areas, d) hypoventilation, e) decrease in FRC.

13. The diffusing capacity for CO in patients with uncomplicated asthma is typically: a) low, b) normal, c) high.

14. An inhaled foreign body most frequently enters: a) left lung, b) right lung, c) no preference.

CHAPTER 5

1. The type 2 epithelial cell a) provides most of the structural support for the normal alveolar wall, b) can multiply and line a damaged alveolar wall, c) can transform into a type 1 epithelial cell, d) secretes surfactant, e) has a very active metabolism.

2. Histological changes in diffuse interstitial pulmonary fibrosis may include: a) infiltration of the alveolar wall with lymphocytes and plasma cells, b) increase in collagen in the interstitial space, c) possible progression to "honeycomb lung," d) sometimes a cellular exudate within the alveoli, e) increased size of the pulmonary capillary bed.

3. Features of diffuse interstitial pulmonary fibrosis typically include: a) dyspnea, especially on exercise, b) prominent cough productive of copious purulent sputum, c) hemoptysis, d) crepitations in both lungs, e) radiologic changes.

4. Pulmonary function tests in diffuse interstitial pulmonary fibrosis typically show: a) low $FEV_{1.0}$, b) low VC, c) low $FEV_{1.0}/FVC\%$, d) low TLC, e) increased airway resistance (related to lung volume).

5. The hypoxemia of a patient with diffuse interstitial pulmonary fibrosis: a) typically worsens on exercise, b) is chiefly caused by $\dot{V}_A/\dot{Q}$ inequality, c) may be partly caused by diffusion impairment, d) is usually associated with CO_2 retention, e) may be worse during exercise than would otherwise be the case because of the abnormally small increase in the cardiac output.

6. Possible factors contributing to the high ventilation during exercise in a patient with diffuse interstitial pulmonary fibrosis include: a) hypoxic stimulation of peripheral chemoreceptors, b) stimulation of intrapulmonary stretch receptors, c) stimulation of central chemoreceptors by an increased arterial P_{CO_2}, d) use of abnormally high tidal volumes.

7. The diffusing capacity for CO in a patient with diffuse interstitial lung disease: a) is typically substantially reduced, b) shows an abnormally small rise during exercise, c) is reduced partly by thickening of the blood gas barrier, d) is reduced partly because of obliteration of pulmonary capillaries, e) falls only very late in the disease.

8. Features of Farmer's Lung include: a) hypersensitivity to spores in moldy hay, b) histological changes primarily in the airways rather than the alveoli, c) restrictive pattern of pulmonary function late in the disease, d) variable amounts or airway obstruction shortly after exposure to the antigen.

9. The following can lead to interstitial pulmonary fibrosis: a) paraquat ingestion, b) oxygen poisoning, c) cigarette smoking, d) radiation to the lung, e) administration of the drug busulfan.

10. Pneumothorax a) may occur spontaneously in apparently fit young adults, b) is usually gradually absorbed in the absence of treatment, c) when present in the tension form is a medical emergency, d) may occur as a complication of mechanical ventilation, e) increases VC.

11. Pulmonary function tests in severe scoliosis typically show: a) an increased FRC, b) hypoxemia, c) a high work of breathing, d) increased pulmonary artery pressure.

CHAPTER 6

1. Factors determining the movement of fluid across the walls of pulmonary capillaries include: a) the hydrostatic pressure in the interstitial space, b) the colloid osmotic pressure of the interstitial fluid, c) the permeability of endothelial cells to water and crystalloids, d) the capillary hydrostatic pressure.

2. In the earliest stages of pulmonary edema: a) fluid tracks through the interstitial space to the perivascular and peribronchial spaces, b) there is an increase in lung lymph flow, c) fluid floods alveoli one by one, d) interstitial hydrostatic pressure probably rises, e) cuffs of fluid collect around the small arteries and veins.

3. When edema fluid is present in the airways: a) hypoxemia occurs as a result of shunts, b) the alveoli which contain fluid become overexpanded, c) frothing of the fluid may occur because of the presence of surfactant, d) during positive pressure ventilation the fluid is moved peripherally.

4. Increased permeability of pulmonary capillaries can be caused by: a) inhaled chlorine gas, b) circulating endotoxin, c) oxygen poisoning, d) aspirin poisoning, e) radiation to the lung.

5. High-altitude pulmonary edema a) is probably caused by an increased capillary permeability as a result of the hypoxia, b) is commonest in people

who acclimatize for long periods, c) is a trivial condition needing no treatment, d) may be related to the high pulmonary artery pressures caused by hypoxic vasoconstriction, e) is best treated by moderate exercise.

6. Severe pulmonary edema with alveolar filling causes: a) reduced lung compliance, b) increased airway resistance, c) hypoxemia which may persist during O_2 breathing, d) rapid shallow respirations.

7. The formation of venous thrombi is favored by: a) dehydration, b) congestive heart failure, c) anemia, d) use of oral contraceptives, e) pregnancy.

8. Presenting features of pulmonary embolism often include: a) pleuritic pain, b) hemoptysis, c) tachycardia, d) pleural friction rub, e) large opacity on the chest radiograph.

9. Moderately large pulmonary emboli often cause: a) arterial hypoxemia, b) increased physiologic dead space, c) some rise in pulmonary artery pressure, d) decreased lung elastic recoil, e) decreased airway resistance.

10. Cor pulmonale: a) may complicate long-standing chronic obstructive lung disease, b) always results in a reduced cardiac output, c) may occur in advanced restrictive lung disease, d) causes neck vein engorgement, e) causes ankle edema.

CHAPTER 7

1. Carbon monoxide a) is the most abundant pollutant in urban atmospheres by weight, b) comes chiefly from power stations and industrial plants, c) is a component of cigarette smoke, d) in the concentrations existing on some freeways, can impair mental skills, e) reduces the P_{O_2} of arterial blood.

2. Inhaled cigarette smoke a) increases the risk of bronchial carcinoma, b) increases the risk of coronary heart disease, c) reduces airway resistance, d) stimulates the autonomic nervous system, e) can raise the blood level of carboxyhemoglobin to 10%.

3. Concerning the deposition of aerosols in the lung: a) many of the largest particles are removed by impaction in the nose and nasopharynx, b) many of the smallest particles (<1 μ) penetrate to the alveoli, c) many inhaled small particles (0.5 μ) are exhaled on the next expiration, d) the small airways are a favored site for sedimentation, e) deposition is reduced on exercise.

4. In the mucociliary system: a) the mucus comes only from goblet cells lining the bronchial epithelium, b) the cilia beat intermittently about 10 times/min, c) the mucous film normally moves at about 1 mm/min in the trachea, d) the mucous film is probably abnormal in asthma, e) the cilia can be paralyzed by inhaled cigarette smoke.

5. Alveolar macrophages a) engulf foreign particles which deposit in the alveoli, b) can migrate to the mucociliary escalator, c) can be killed by ingested silica, d) may kill ingested bacteria before these are removed from the alveoli, e) secrete alveolar surfactant.

6. Simple coal miner's pneumoconiosis a) is a direct result of inhaling large amounts of coal dust, b) may progress to "progressive massive fibrosis,"

c) typically causes striking cough and dyspnea at rest, d) causes a fine mottling on the chest radiograph, e) cause a marked reduction in the diffusing capacity for CO.

7. With regard to asbestosis: a) this may occur in men employed in pipe-lagging, b) it can cause diffuse interstitial fibrosis, c) it is associated with an increased incidence of bronchial carcinoma, d) mesothelioma may occur long after light exposure, e) asbestos fibers in the sputum can often be recognized.

8. Concerning byssinosis a) it is caused by exposure to wool fibers, b) it causes wheezing and dyspnea, c) pulmonary function tests show a reduced $FEV_{1.0}$, VC, and $FEV_{1.0}/FVC\%$, d) the symptoms are worst when the patient returns to work after a 2- or 3-day absence, e) the disease progresses to diffuse interstitial pulmonary fibrosis.

9. Bronchial carcinoma a) the disease has a higher prevalence in urban as opposed to rural communities, b) the disease is commoner in males than females, c) the specific carcinogenic agent in cigarette smoke is known, d) pulmonary function tests are important in the early detection of the disease, e) a carcinoma is always visible on a good chest radiograph.

10. In cystic fibrosis a) the disease is confined to the lungs, b) affected children invariably die before the age of 15, c) finger clubbing does not occur, d) analysis of the sweat is useful in screening, e) uneven ventilation is an early abnormality of pulmonary function.

CHAPTER 8

1. Severe hypoxemia can cause: a) tachycardia, b) lactic acidemia, c) retinal hemorrhages, d) mental clouding, e) proteinuria.

2. CO_2 retention causes: a) acidosis, b) reduced cerebral blood flow, c) renal retention of bicarbonate, d) mental clouding, e) raised CSF pressure.

3. A patient was admitted to hospital with an acute exacerbation of chronic lung disease. When given 100% O_2 his arterial P_{CO_2} increased from 50 to 80 mm Hg. Likely causes were: a) increase in airway resistance, b) release of hypoxic vasoconstriction in poorly ventilated areas of lung, c) depression of ventilation, d) depression of cardiac output, e) reduced levels of 2,3-DPG in the blood.

4. Acidosis in respiratory failure is likely to be increased by: a) depression of ventilation, b) exacerbation of a chest infection, c) peripheral circulatory failure, d) renal retention of bicarbonate, e) administration of morphine.

5. Features of the adult respiratory distress syndrome include: a) severe hypoxemia, b) severe CO_2 retention, c) reduced lung compliance, d) reduced FRC, e) large shunt.

6. Features of the infant respiratory distress syndrome include: a) patchy hemorrhagic edema and atelectasis, b) absence of pulmonary surfactant, c) severe hypoxemia, d) large shunt, e) increased risk in premature infants.

7. An exacerbation of bronchitis in a patient with advanced chronic obstructive lung disease typically: a) increases airway resistance, b) causes wors-

ening of $\dot{V}_A/\dot{Q}$ relationships, c) causes marked leucocytosis and pyrexia, d) may result in CO_2 retention, e) is generally well tolerated without specific treatment.

CHAPTER 9

1. A young man who was previously well was admitted to the emergency room with barbiturate poisoning which caused severe hypoventilation. When he was given 50% O_2 to breathe there was no change in his arterial P_{CO_2}. Approximately how much would his arterial P_{O_2} (mm Hg) be expected to rise? a) 25, b) 50, c) 75, d) 100, e) 200.

2. When a patient with severe $\dot{V}_A/\dot{Q}$ inequality was given 80% O_2 to breathe, it was found that his arterial P_{O_2} rose to only 300 mm Hg. Factors which might have contributed to this unexpectedly low level include: a) presence of lung units with very low $\dot{V}_A/\dot{Q}$ values, b) atelectasis of low $\dot{V}_A/\dot{Q}$ units as a result of the high inspired P_{O_2}, c) relief of hypoxic vasoconstriction in poorly ventilated areas, d) loss of alveolar surface area resulting in a low diffusing capacity.

3. A patient with congenital heart disease has a right-to-left shunt and an arterial P_{O_2} of 60 mm Hg during air breathing. When he is given 100% O_2, you would expect his arterial P_{O_2} to rise: a) not at all, b) less than 10 mm Hg, c) more than 10 mm Hg, d) to about 600 mm Hg.

4. A patient with severe CO poisoning was given an exchange transfusion of stored blood. Measurement of his O_2 dissociation curve showed a marked reduction in P_{50}. Likely causative factors were: a) arterial CO_2 retention, b) residual CO level in the blood, c) abnormally low concentration of 2,3-DPG in the transfused red cells, d) reduced arterial pH, e) mild pyrexia.

5. Advantages of nasal cannulas for O_2 administration include: a) they can be worn comfortably for long periods, b) inspired O_2 concentrations of up to 60% are readily obtained, c) the inspired O_2 concentration is accurately known, d) the inspired P_{CO_2} does not rise.

6. O_2 masks based on the Venturi principle are useful because: a) they give inspired O_2 concentrations of up to 60%, b) the inspired O_2 concentration is well controlled, c) the inspired P_{CO_2} is low, d) the inspired O_2 concentration increases automatically if the ventilation rises.

7. Uses of hyperbaric O_2 include treatment of: a) adult respiratory distress syndrome, b) severe CO poisoning, c) gas gangrene infections, d) spontaneous pneumothorax, e) some malignant tumors by radiotherapy.

8. Intermittent O_2 therapy may be dangerous in the treatment of respiratory failure because: a) the arterial P_{CO_2} rises rapidly when the O_2 is stopped, b) the arterial P_{O_2} falls to very low levels when the O_2 is stopped, c) the pulmonary artery pressure rises to high levels, d) systemic hypertension may occur.

9. In pulmonary O_2 toxicity, the first histological changes probably occur in: a) type 1 epithelial cells, b) type 2 epithelial cells, c) interstitium, d) capillary endothelial cells, e) alveolar macrophages.

10. Lung units with low $\dot{V}_A/\dot{Q}$ ratios may collapse when high concentrations

of O_2 are inhaled for 1 hr because: a) pulmonary surfactant is inactivated, b) O_2 toxicity causes intra-alveolar edema, c) gas is taken up by the blood faster than it enters the unit by ventilation, d) interstitial edema around the small airways causes airway closure.

CHAPTER 10

1. A tracheostomy tube a) facilitates the removal of secretions by suction, b) provides a port for mechanical ventilation, c) can be used to bypass a region of upper airway obstruction, d) increases the anatomical dead space.
2. Constant-volume ventilators typically a) do not require electrical power, b) are small, compact, and portable, c) provide a nearly constant tidal volume even if lung compliance fails, d) do not allow the respiratory frequency to be changed.
3. In intermittent positive pressure ventilation, a long inspiratory time: a) tends to reduce the regional inequality of ventilation, b) tends to diminish venous return to the thorax, c) tends to reduce FRC, d) in general should be avoided in favor of an inspiratory-expiratory time ratio of less than 1.
4. In the treatment of the adult respiratory distress syndrome the addition of 15 cm water of PEEP typically: a) increases FRC, b) reduces shunt, c) increases alveolar edema, d) increases physiological dead space, e) tends to reduce venous return to the thorax.
5. Mechanical ventilation tends to reduce cardiac output: a) because it reduces pulmonary vascular resistance, b) because it reduces the pressure difference responsible for returning venous blood to the thorax, c) especially if the circulating blood volume is abnormally low, d) with positive pressure ventilators but not with tank respirators, e) but even if it does this cannot reduce tissue P_{O_2}.
6. Hazards of mechanical ventilation include: a) pneumothorax, b) raised CSF pressure, c) interstitial emphysema, d) pulmonary infection, e) retinal hemorrhage.

Answers

CHAPTER 1

1. a) Volume exhaled in 1 sec by a forced expiration from full inspiration. b) Middle half (by volume) of a forced expiration from full inspiration, divided by its duration.
2. d.
3. Alveolar minus intrapleural pressure (approximately).
4. a, b, c, d
5. b, c.
6. b.
7. a.
8. a, b.
9. b, d.
10. d.

CHAPTER 2

1. c, d.
2. b, d.
3. c.
4. b, c.
5. P_{O_2} which the lung would have if there were no $\dot{V}_A/\dot{Q}$ inequality and the respiratory change ratio remained the same.
6. $V_D/V_T = (P_a - P_E)/P_a$.
7. Because of the different shapes of the O_2 and CO_2 dissociation curves.
8. About 7.2

9. Mixed respiratory and metabolic acidosis.
10. a, c.

CHAPTER 3

1. a, b, e.
2. a, b.
3. a, d.
4. a, b, c.
5. a, c.
6. Increased elimination of CO_2 following the liberation of lactic acid from hypoxic muscles, and excessive hyperventilation caused by stimulation of intrapulmonary receptors (?J).
7. a, b, e.

CHAPTER 4

1. Disease characterized by enlargement of air spaces distal to the terminal bronchioles, with destruction of their walls.
2. a) Upper zone, b) lower zone, c) no preference, or possibly lower zone.
3. b, c.
4. Ratio of thickness of mucous glands to bronchial wall.
5. b, c, f.
6. None.
7. a) Almost normal, b) displaced to right with reduced slope.

8. d.
9. a, b, c, d.
10. a, b, c, d.
11. a, c, e.
12. c.
13. b or c.
14. b.

CHAPTER 5

1. b, c, d, e.
2. a, b, c, d.
3. a, d, e.
4. a, b, d.
5. a, b, c, e.
6. a, b.
7. a, b, c, d.
8. a, c, d.
9. a, b, d, e.
10. a, b, c, d.
11. b, c, d.

CHAPTER 6

1. a, b, d.
2. a, b, d, e.
3. a, c, d.
4. a, b, c, e.
5. d.
6. a, b, c, d.
7. a, b, d, e.
8. a, b, c, d.
9. a, b, c.
10. a, c, d, e.

CHAPTER 7

1. a, c, d.
2. a, b, d, e.
3. a, b, c, d.

4. d, e.
5. a, b, c, d.
6. a, b, d.
7. All.
8. b, c, d.
9. a, b.
10. d, e.

CHAPTER 8

1. All.
2. a, c, d, e.
3. b, c.
4. a, b, c, e.
5. a, c, d, e.
6. All.
7. a, b, d.

CHAPTER 9

1. e.
2. a, b, c.
3. c.
4. b, c.
5. a, d.
6. b, c.
7. b, c, e.
8. b.
9. d.
10. c.

CHAPTER 10

1. a, b, c.
2. c.
3. a, b, d.
4. a, b, d, e.
5. b, c.
6. a, c, d.

Index

Cilia, 142
Clearance of deposited particles from
 lung, 141
Closing volume, 17–18, 47
 age dependence, 17
 increase in early disease, 18
 mechanism, 17
Coal workers' pneumoconiosis, 140,
 143–145
 clinical features, 144
 histology, 140
 progressive massive fibrosis, 145
Collagen diseases causing interstitial
 fibrosis, 107
Collateral ventilation, 16–17
Compensated respiratory acidosis, 38
Compliance, 44, see also Lung
 compliance
Constant pressure ventilators, 189
Constant volume ventilators, 188
Continuous positive airway pressure,
 196
Control of ventilation, 48–50
 in chronic obstructive lung disease,
 49
 interpretation, 49
 measurement, 48
Cor pulmonale, 132
Corticosteroids in asthma, 84
Critical ventilation-perfusion ratio,
 185
Cromolyn sodium, 85
Crushed chest, 26
Cuirass ventilator, 192, 201
Curschmann's spirals, 81
Cyanosis, 21
Cyclic AMP, 81
Cystic fibrosis, 152–153
 clinical features, 153
 pathology, 152
 pulmonary function, 153

Dead space, increased by mechanical
 ventilation, 196
Diaphragm fatigue, 162
Diffuse interstitial fibrosis, 26, see
 also Diffuse interstitial
 pulmonary fibrosis
 effect on lung volume, 43

Diffuse interstitial pulmonary
 fibrosis, 96–103
 arterial Pco_2 in, 100
 cause of hypoxemia in, 100
 changes on exercise in, 102
 clinical features, 96
 control of ventilation in, 103
 diffusing capacity in, 101
 diffusion impairment, 99
 distribution of ventilation-perfusion
 ratios, 100
 gas exchange, 98
 histology, 97
 lung volumes, 98
 pathology, 96
 pulmonary function, 97
 radiographic appearance, 96
 ventilatory capacity, 98
Diffusing capacity, 39–41
 causes of reduction, 40
 interpretation, 41
 measurement, 40
Diffusion
 in diffuse interstitial pulmonary
 fibrosis, 100
 in peripheral lung units, 16
Diffusion impairment, 22, 26, 173
 effect of exercise, 26
 response of hypoxemia to added O_2,
 29
 role in causing hypoxemia, 27
2,3-Diphosphoglycerate, 21, 177
Distortion, of lung, by gravity, 17
Distribution of blood flow, 53
Distribution of ventilation, 54
Domiciliary oxygen, 179
Dynamic compliance, 47
Dynamic compression of airways, 9,
 47
Dyspnea, 52–53

Edema, pulmonary, see Pulmonary
 edema
Elastic properties, of lung, 43–45
 interpretation, 44
 measurement, 43
Elastic recoil, of lung, 44
Embolism, pulmonary, see Pulmonary
 embolism